HOSPICE AND MINISTRY

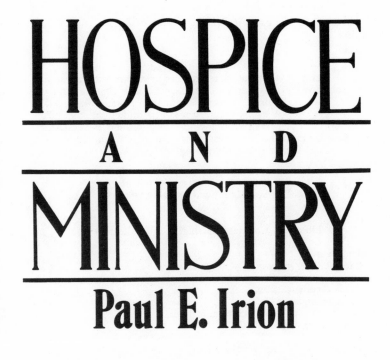

HOSPICE
A N D
MINISTRY

Paul E. Irion

ABINGDON PRESS

NASHVILLE

HOSPICE AND MINISTRY

Copyright © 1988 by Abingdon Press

This book is printed on acid-free paper.

Library of Congress Cataloging-in-Publication Data

Irion, Paul E.
  Hospice and ministry.

  Bibliography: p.
  Includes index.
  1. Church work with the terminally ill.
2. Hospice care. I. Title.
BV4460.6.I75   1988   259'.4   87-33656
ISBN 0-687-17490-2 (pbk.: alk. paper)

ISBN 0-687-17490-2

Excerpt from *When a Friend Is Dying* by Edward F. Dobihal, Jr., and Charles
William Stewart, copyright © 1984 assigned to Edward F. Dobihal and
Charles W. Stewart; used by permission of authors.

MANUFACTURED BY THE PARTHENON PRESS AT
NASHVILLE, TENNESSEE, UNITED STATES OF AMERICA

To the professional staff
and volunteers in
Hospice of Lancaster County,
who make caring real.

_____

CONTENTS

INTRODUCTION

This is not so much a book about hospice as it is about the pastoral care given in the hospice setting. It is based on the shared experiences of more than sixty pastors who have ministered to parishioners who were hospice patients.

We are concerned here not simply with techniques for dealing with the terminally ill and their families. This study is centered on the hospice philosophy, a philosophy that shapes the attitudes and actions of those who give hospice care. Since the pastor is often a significant contributor to such care, this philosophy can have a profound effect upon the pastor's work as well. Many professionals have found that working in hospice has caused them to rethink and restructure some of their approaches.

I have been interested in this project since early contact in 1969 with St. Christopher's Hospice in London. I was actively involved in founding Hospice of Lancaster County (Pennsylvania) and have seen it grow into a highly effective community agency with a staff of eighteen professionals and fifty-four volunteers, caring for 255 families during the past year. For a year I served on a volunteer basis as Pastoral Care

Coordinator, becoming familiar with the spiritual needs seen in many patients and families and with the ways in which parish pastors worked with them.

In order to broaden my study, I contacted one hundred other hospices from the membership of the National Hospice Organization and asked them to give me names of parish pastors who had demonstrated to their staffs particular effectiveness as pastoral caregivers. I received the names of more than a hundred pastors.

A questionnaire was sent to these pastors, exploring in detail ways in which they thought their ministry to the terminally ill had been affected by their work with parishioners who were hospice patients. I asked them to compare their ministry to the terminally ill in hospice programs and in non-hospice hospital settings, with particular reference to what I had defined (but not delineated) in the questionnaire as specific attributes of the hospice approach.

They were asked, for example, in which setting did they, as pastors, feel more a part of the caregiving team? In which was there more involvement with the patient and the family? In which setting was there more apparent acceptance of approaching death? More conversation with the family about death? In which setting was there more effective facilitating of the grieving process? and so on.

Pastors were also asked to comment in detail on which aspects of the hospice approach contributed to their pastoral care and which aspects limited their helpfulness. They were asked to describe as fully as possible their last visit to a hospice patient.

More than 50 percent of the pastors queried responded in considerable detail, helpfully describing the pastoral care they were able to give to dying hospice patients and their families. I then selected about thirty pastors for personal interviews, in which their experiences were explored more fully.

It should be pointed out that anecdotal case material has come from a number of hospice programs and has been disguised in non-essential details to maintain confidentiality.

I am grateful to the hospice staff members and parish pastors who cooperated in making this study possible. These endeavors are part of the constant commitment of hospice workers to ask, How can we strengthen our caregiving?

CHAPTER 1

HOSPICE AND THE PARISH PASTOR

When hospices got started in some communities, the reaction of some physicians was, "I've been dealing with terminal patients for a long time. I don't do so badly. Hospice isn't really needed here." It is possible that some clergy reacted in similar fashion. Recent history demonstrates, however, that hospice has made a difference. New attitudes and innovative approaches to the terminally ill have emerged from hospice operations, which are having a salutary effect on many helping disciplines.

Henri Nouwen applied the notion of caring in the absence of cure to working with the aged.[1] It is no less applicable to hospice and the care of the terminally ill, for aging and terminality have a good deal in common.

As the wonders of medical treatment have multiplied, it has been easy to correlate caring and curing. When cure is no longer possible, it is almost automatic to say, "There is nothing more that we can do." We have failed to recognize that there is always something that can be done. Care can be given, even in the absence of cure.

Hospice institutionalized that option. It stands as a strong reminder that there is a great deal that can be done for those for whom cure is no longer a relevant issue. Hospice has brought this insight to a broad spectrum of caregivers, including the clergy.

Hospice Made a Difference for Its Patients

Hospices in Great Britain, which were the inspiration for the development of hospices in the United States, were in-patient institutions with some care given in the patient's home prior to admission to the facility. When hospices began to be formed in the U.S., new forms and designs were strongly encouraged. Only a few clearly modeled themselves after their British prototypes and became freestanding in-patient facilities only for the care of the terminally ill, with supportive home care. Some others developed as services within established hospitals, most often with supportive home care. The majority of American hospices developed as programs emphasizing home care, supported by the possibility of in-patient admission. If hospice concepts are thoroughly followed, the location of patient care is of secondary importance. However, there are some unique elements, as we shall see, in the home care component.

Like its medieval forebear, hospice has offered refuge to those who are exhausted and gravely ill. It has provided a support system that enables a way of dying by living to the fullest in the months and weeks that remain. It has enabled patients and families to deal together with this crisis that involves them all. It has used methods of medication that enable most patients to be free of oppressive pain. It has expressed a concern for all facets of the patient's life—a holistic approach to living and dying.

It is the purpose of this book to explore in detail the ways in which pastoral care of the terminally ill has been affected by the development of hospice. The common design for hospices, which has emerged during this period of rapid expansion, includes the provision of pastoral care for those who want it. The major accrediting systems (the National Hospice Organization and the Joint Commission on Accreditation of Hospitals) require that hospices make some provision for spiritual care.

Hospice does many things intentionally that may or may not happen in the care of the terminally ill in other settings. It does not have a monopoly on these approaches to the dying patient and his or her family, but it does have a structure which includes them by design rather than happenstance. These elements have implications for pastoral care. They include a holistic approach, openness in dealing with death, pain control, the family as the unit of care, a home care setting (in many but not all instances), self-determination for the patient and his or her family in decision making, a blend of professional and lay caregivers, and sustained bereavement aftercare.

Hospice Made a Difference to Pastors

In any activity that goes beyond the purely mechanical, there is an integral connection between the practice and the practitioner. Help is not discreetly separated from the helper. So the unique dimensions of hospice care will affect both pastoral care and the pastor as a person. Liston Mills suggests of hospice: "As important as this institutional development is, I do not see it as a solution to our common problem [dealing with death]. That solution must come in the lives of professional practitioners, doctors, ministers, nurses, social workers, etc."[2]

Interviews with a number of pastors who have been ministering in hospice settings give personal testimony to the ways in which they feel hospice has changed them as persons. They said: "Hospice has made me more of a person." "Hospice has added more compassion to my ministry." "Working with hospice patients has filled me with a lot more pain, pain that hasn't all been released." "Hospice has helped me work with my own mortality." "Hospice made it easier for me to express myself as a feeling person." "I have become more willing to let someone be dependent on me."

Others expressed the effect it had on their ministries: "Hospice patients helped me realize that I don't have all the answers." "My preaching is much more sensitive, more 'in the kitchen' where the real issues of life are." "I do not trust people who want stereotyped support. I work with the impulse to grapple."

Resisting the temptation to overly romanticize the fruits of participating in hospice, we must recognize certain dangers. It is possible to use professional techniques of ministry, such as praying or administering the sacraments, while keeping one's distance from the patient. It is possible to theologize about death and suffering in the abstract, without becoming involved with the dying. There is nothing wrong with praying, administering the sacraments, or theologizing—as long as they do not become substitutes for dealing personally with the dying patient or for confronting one's own mortality.

In the Christian tradition, there has always been a concern to minister to those who are dying. Pastoral responses have run the gamut from pressing for deathbed conversions to being a supportive presence in the final hours of life. As modern pastoral care has been informed by the growing literature on death and dying, ministry to the dying and grieving has begun to blend in psychological and theological insights.

Recognition of the facts that life is fleeting and death is inevitable brings many persons face to face with ultimate questions. They reach out to what they regard as enduring values, to find some meaning in these profound experiences. Some are exploring the dimensions of a new experience; others are fearful and stressed. Either instance constitutes a spiritual concern.

Definitions of Spiritual Care

Defining spirituality is not an easy task. Not only is it intangible and mysterious, it is also subject to highly individualized understanding.

Some definitions are dualistic, organized by a differentiation of physical and spiritual orders of reality. Some definitions are explicitly theological, dealing with the individual's relationship with God or the transcendent. Still other definitions are functional: Spirituality is a way of describing the organizing center of one's life—that which brings unity to the diverse elements of experience.

This latter definition will be used here for two reasons. It describes an essential function of human existence, and it does so in a way that reflects the uniqueness of each person's experience. Spirituality refers to a quality of life in which there is a cohesiveness, an integrity, a sense of wholeness.

Some people will describe this unitary quality in terms of a theological belief system: as living with God, being in Christ, hoping for life after death. Some will use more abstract terms: that which gives meaning and purpose to life. Rather than insisting upon a normative understanding, effective pastoral care of the dying hospice patient and family will be able to respond to the way in which these persons define the spiritual, explicitly or implicitly.

Most of the work that has been done on spiritual care in the hospice setting avoids giving narrow definitions. To describe spiritual care, Beresford uses phrases like "helping to bring acceptance into the life of a dying patient . . . helping to facilitate the exploration and discovery of meaning . . . communicating God's love to people in need . . . helping patients explore their life stories . . . encouraging . . . to live for the present moment . . . being a friend."[3] Munley describes spiritual caregiving as "the capacity to enter into the world of the other and to respond with feeling . . . touching another at a level that is deeper than ideological and doctrinal differences."[4] Davidson writes of "stories, symbols, rituals—which allow mourners to move from the fragmenting, alienating and disorienting consequences of change to a renewed sense of wholeness."[5]

The common themes of these definitions are relatedness, getting in touch with that which brings wholeness, and meaning. Far less attention is given to more traditional understandings of preparing people to die, to deathbed conversions, and to getting people to assent to particular theological propositions.

There are a number of reasons why hospices have found it difficult to define pastoral or spiritual care in very specific terms.

It is inevitable that the pluralism of American society will have an impact on the way hospices regard pastoral care, especially since such care has become virtually mandated as a part of hospice programs. Dedicated to serving the entire community, hospices deal with people of all backgrounds: socio-economic, ethnic, religious. In the light of that diverse clientele, to insist on having spiritual caregiving as a component of hospices requires a very broad definition of spiritual care.

Because hospice by its very nature is focused on the individuality of the patient and his or her family, it feels a responsibility to reflect and protect the patient's beliefs or lack of belief. There is an inherent resistance to pressing a particular belief stance on anyone. Caregivers are so highly motivated to care for individuals on their (i.e., the individuals') own terms that they refrain from pressing their belief systems on patients and families.

The standards which are advanced by accrediting bodies are responsive to the pluralistic situation in which we live. These standards are framed in language that permits broad latitude in defining or describing spiritual care.

Hospices, with some justification due to bad experiences in the past, have been cautious in establishing close linkage with the religious community. There is some fear of sectarian imperialism, in which a particular religious group would press its views as norms for hospice practice. In the same way, hospices have been frightened off by some pastors who have been strongly judgmental of patients, who have proselytized, who have been rigid in their relationships with patients, or who have presented religious faith in ways that fostered evasive and escapist attitudes.

The difficulties apparent in establishing definitive guidelines of hospice spiritual care may tempt one to the suggestion of Munley:

> Attentiveness to spiritual needs and concerns is a major element of hospice ideology, yet descriptions of the process of spiritual caregiving in American hospices are virtually nonexistent. Should it be assumed that hospices in pluralistic American society need to be sponsored by organized religions in order to deliver spiritual care effectively?[6]

This cannot be seen as the only, or even the most desirable, option. A more helpful solution may be the establishing of closer and more effective working relationships between hospices and the clergy of the community. Pastors serving their own parishioners who are hospice patients are more apt to be closer to common ground with them. However, even here it should not be assumed that churches or congregations are absolutely monolithic in their beliefs. There always has to be sensitive acknowledgment and empathic respect for the varieties of individual interpretation.

Spiritual/Religious Issues of
Hospice Patients and Families

Although room always has to be left for individual differences, there are some spiritual issues that are frequently encountered. These focus largely on exploring the relational ties that give substance to living, on the meanings upon which one stakes one's dedication to the values of life, on developing a sense of self-worth, and on finding strength for coping.

1. Belonging and Relationship

Death is a very isolating experience. It involves the breaking of significant relationships. The dying person becomes aware that even though others are present, only he or she is dying. Some feel abandoned—by medical science, by friends, by God. Some people experience approaching death as a great loneliness.

There is a proper pastoral concern about impending severance of interpersonal relationships. Death is creating an abyss between persons who have lived side by side. Whether this severance refers to disruptions of relationships between persons or to the existential separation that results from the fact that one person is dying in the midst of others who will go on living, the pastor has a concern for bringing peace to those relationships. This may be particularly important to women, for as one hospice caregiver has pointed out, male patients tend to talk about meaning, while female patients more often framed their concerns about relationships. The work of Carol Gilligan would support this observation.[7]

22

Many pastors who have worked with hospice patients indicate that dying patients often voice more concern for their families than for themselves. "What is my illness doing to my family?" is a relatively common query, especially from younger and early middle-age patients who still have dependent family members.

From the time of Tolstoy's *Death of Ivan Ilyitch*, there has been a clearer understanding of the way in which awareness of approaching death can produce a deeper bondedness with oneself, with others, and with the world. Some persons are able to expand their range of emotional expression in such a time, finding a growing capacity to love and to express love. A pastor described a situation in which a hospice patient in the very late stage of her illness called her husband to her bed, hugged him, and told him how much she appreciated the loving care he had been giving. She repeated the same process with her son and daughter, put her head back on her pillow, closed her eyes, and died in a few minutes.

Part of the pastoral task is to help families who are becoming disconnected in this crisis situation. Usually one can see in a family configuration one person who provides a great deal of the family strength. An astute pastor can help a family to reconnect around that person.

Some dying persons experience a sense of abandonment. Their losses are compound, ranging from the loss of relationship to the loss of faith and hope. This produces loneliness and fear, a sense of being cut off and unsupported.

The need to feel a sense of belonging in the context of dying and separation is a focus for pastoral care. Pastors who have ministered to hospice patients said: "People need to feel that God loves them in spite of all this." "In word and deed I try to surround the patient incarnationally with the love of God that can redeem life beyond this suffering." "I do what I can to communicate the trustability of God, of unconditional love."

Sometimes the sense of belonging with God involves feeling forgiven. Patients may assess their lives and feel wanting. They are aware of failures and of wrongs that they have done. They want to talk about the guilt or regret they are feeling. This is the traditional way of expressing the need for reconciliation of a disrupted relationship.

A pastor told of the experience of Jack, a fifty-five-year-old man who had not been involved with the church for thirty years. He had struggled against the thought of dying. He asked the hospice staff to arrange for a pastor to visit. After several visits he asked to receive communion. This service seemed to free him to die, and he did a few hours later.

Others may want to talk about their anger, their feelings of having wronged or been wronged, their doubts. Just as they are fighting with their disease, they may also be acting out a great deal of defiance toward that which they experience as over against them, including God. All of these are poignant efforts to experience a sense of belonging. Some pastors have suggested that less anger persists in hospice patients because as people are encouraged to express their feelings openly, they can get them out and be done with it.

2. Meaning

Part of the spiritual struggle is to find meaning in this experience, even as health is being diminished. Death with dignity is death with meaning. Human beings find it very difficult to encounter death unless some way is found to link it to meaning. Heroism or martyrdom are very pronounced attributions of meaning. Less obvious are interpretations that see death as fitting into a larger plan, as bringing an end to pain or weakness, or as marking the suitable conclusion of a full, rich life.

One of the pastors interviewed put it this way: "It is easy to make contact with the patients' loneliness. Their hunger for meaning comes out into the open if they are given a chance to talk." To be most helpful, meaning is drawn out from the patient, rather than being imposed upon him or her.

It is not at all uncommon for people in the context of approaching death to ask questions. Some of the questions pastors reported having been asked are "What is it like to die?" "Where is God in this process?" "Has my life been significant?" "How does God deal with people who haven't done all they should?" "What is it like to be with God?" According to a number of pastors, more families commonly inquire, "Why him (or her)?" than patients ask, "Why me?"

Such questions have two dimensions. On the one hand, they are the expression of a search for insight; on the other hand, they are expressions of deep feelings: fear, guilt, anger, abandonment. Several hospice pastoral caregivers reported that they interpret "why" questions as expressions of non-acceptance of the process of dying. They find that high-level caring for the patient reduces feelings of dereliction. In their experience, they have seen many hospice patients who have moved beyond the "why" questions that were asked earlier in their experiences of illness.

One does not start with a blank slate. People who have done any thinking at all have a system of meaning, even if only rudimentary, by which they live. They may not have put it into words in any systematic fashion. With some encouragement from the pastor, they can begin to articulate and explore what meaning they are able to find in their present situation.

The pastor who works with hospice patients will encounter questions—difficult, unavoidable, unanswerable questions. It is glib either to provide ready answers or to imply that a question should not be asked. The constructive pastoral response is to acknowledge the importance of a question to the person and to be open to talking about it. Such questions are "lived with" in the fullest sense of the word.

Finding the "real question" is very important. Often there are two levels in a query. There is an apparent request for some information, and there is, possibly, a deep concern which motivates the question. Sometimes questions about life after death, reunion with family members, and final judgment may represent only information seeking, but they may also be ways of expressing a need to deal with guilt or with the fear of separation from loved ones. The pastor who limits pastoral concern to dealing with the informational level, answering questions, will relate to only a portion of the parishioner's concerns.

The pastor is an active part of the pastoral relationship and of the quest for meaning. Like all thoughtful humans and usually more than most, the pastor has thought about these issues. Even though the pastor is thoroughly committed to the hospice ideal of dealing with the patient in terms of his or her spirituality and of not pressing personal views on the patient, there is not a total prohibition of expressing one's own views. If the patient asks the pastor, "What do you think?" it is possible and helpful to share one's own grappling with the questions. This needs to be done in a context of intellectual humility, acknowledging that these are personal beliefs rather than "correct answers" to metaphysical questions.

There are times when a pastor sees the patient or

family finding in their religious understandings a basis for denying what is going on in their lives. People will put singular confidence in a miraculous reversal of their illness, as in the case of Peter, who, when his physician indicated that chemotherapy was not being effective and should be discontinued, began to assert that he could feel Jesus shrinking his tumor. Without necessarily supporting that perception, the understanding pastor can certainly respond empathically to the patient's reaching out for something hopeful. The range of things that can be hoped for becomes an appropriate focus of conversation.

Sometimes the pastor faces a similar dilemma when the patient begins to articulate answers that give evidence of being counterproductive. Suppose, for example, that the patient begins to answer the "why" question with an assertion that the illness is a punishment from a wrathful God. One does not argue with that perception or scold the person for thinking that way. The pastor accepts the pain of the patient and suggests that there may be several ways of understanding the situation. Mills writes of such instances:

> [The pastor] simply stands and points. His standing with the person shows him as mortal, too, caught in the same suffering, facing the same death, in need of the same comfort . . . His pointing is to the source of his faith, the God who beckons us to trust that covenant and hope abide.[8]

3. Self-worth

Meaning and a sense of personal worth are closely interdependent. One cannot feel self-esteem without a sense of meaning, and one cannot find meaning in life if it has no value.

In a society that highly prizes vitality, illness can be very demeaning and dying the ultimate indignity. One of the spiritual needs of the dying person is for affirmation of self-worth. This is one of the essential ingredients of what has come to be called "quality of life."

One might wonder how self-worth can be communicated to one who is living out human mortality in dramatic fashion. There are two ways in which this might be attempted. On one hand, there might be a denial of mortality, a deflection of the impact of death with religious teaching of immortality. On the other hand, there might be an open and honest sharing of mortality. It is not accidental that many people who work in hospice programs state that they are able to deal more honestly with their own mortality through their relationships with dying persons. This is not merely empathy, but an actual sharing of the awareness of mortality. For the dying to be cared for deeply by those who share in their mortality is a way of communicating self-worth.

> Intimacy with the dying and those close to them inevitably brings us to a confrontation with impoverishment . . . which comes from recognizing the foolishness, impotence, and mortality of any one creature's life reflected against the vastness of universe. We can only bear, at any stage in life, to see a little of this poverty that distinguishes human life. The dying, however, are immersed in it—the signs of their creatureliness and finiteness surround them on every side, as they sink into the commonness of death. It must be accepted, and it can be more readily accepted if those closest to the patient can share their own impoverishment.[9]

A pastor can support the self-worth of the dying person by helping the person to be actively involved in his or her situation, by participating in decisions and by continuing in relationships; all the elements that are sustained in hospice care. For a person to see that dying is an active rather than a passive process can enhance self-esteem. Dobihal and Stewart point this out very helpfully:

> When the person who is dying hears "What is it you want?" and receives care in such a way that he or she can believe those words are important, it is spiritually uplifting. It conveys the message that the person is still important, still of great worth.[10]

This is part of the reality testing in which the hospice patient is involved. It proceeds on several levels. The person tests the reality of the situation of dying. The person also tests the reality of the effect of that dying upon his or her selfhood. Spiritual care offers the assurance that one can die with an intact sense of self-worth.

4. Coping

One pastor described hospice patients as "trying to define some kind of *scenario* to live out." This suggests that they are looking for those things that will enable them to accomplish a smooth transition from health and life to illness and death. Their disease makes them feel vulnerable and powerless at times; they feel they need to learn to cope with their unfolding situations.

Only as they are able to feel a measure of control over the circumstances of their lives at this point will they be able to cope. Of course, they quickly become aware that they cannot control whether or not they will die. But they can have a measure of control over the way they will die. The pastor has an opportunity to help them understand the possibilities that are before them and to support them in deciding which of those possibilities will be most fruitful for them.

The first thing they need is the *desire* to cope. Illness

29

may have produced so much passivity in some that they feel incapable of coping. The pastor can help them explore ways in which they have coped with stressful crises in the past. They can be reminded of resources to help them cope: relationship, personal values, faith.

There is a subtle selectivity in the way a pastor responds to the religious reflections of the patient or family member. While acknowledging what the person has said, it is possible to emphasize themes that will assist coping. The pastor may well emphasize imagery of the nurturing, caring parent rather than the punitive one, or may stress the mercy rather than the judgment of God. Such selectivity is justified, particularly if the pastor can communicate an awareness of the deep feelings and concerns which underlie the words of the parishioner.

Because the sense of vulnerability does not leave, there needs to be regular reinforcement of the coping processes that are operating. There has to be a new openness to possibilities and choices, as time passes.

Summary

In these various ways a pastor has the opportunity to respond to deep spiritual need in the hospice patient. The pastoral relationship becomes an avenue for supporting the patient in the quest for a sense of belonging, for meaning, and for a feeling of self-worth. As we shall see later, the hospice setting supports pastoral care in dealing with these needs.

NOTES

1. Henri J. M. Nouwen, *Care and the Elderly* (New York: The Ministers and Missionaries Benefit Board of the American Baptist Churches).

2. Liston O. Mills, "Issues for the Clergy in the Care of the Dying and Bereaved," in *Dying and Death*, ed. David Barton (Baltimore: Williams & Wilkins, 1977), p. 205.

3. Larry Beresford, "Spiritual Care in Hospice," *California Hospice Report* 2, no. 7 (Dec. 1984): 4-5.

4. Anne Munley, *The Hospice Alternative* (New York: Basic Books, 1983), p. 268.

5. Glen W. Davidson, ed., *The Hospice: Development and Administration*, 2nd ed. (Washington: Hemisphere Publishing Corp., 1985), p. 146.

6. Munley, *The Hospice Alternative*, p. 228.

7. Carol Gilligan, *In a Different Voice: Psychological Theory and Women's Development* (Cambridge: Harvard University Press, 1982).

8. Mills, "Issues for the Clergy," p. 207.

9. Paul S. Dawson, "Reflections of a Hospice Chaplain," in *A Hospice Handbook*, ed. Michael Hamilton and Helen Reid (Grand Rapids: Eerdmans, 1980), p. 70.

10. Edward F. Dobihal, Jr., and Charles William Stewart, *When a Friend Is Dying* (Nashville: Abingdon Press, 1984), p. 33.

CHAPTER 2

THE HOLISTIC APPROACH OF HOSPICE: THE SETTING FOR PASTORAL CARE

The importation of hospice from England in 1970 and its rapid spread across the United States in the decade that followed was brought about by the activities of countless individuals and groups who wanted hospices for their communities. These early proponents of the hospice movement were community leaders from a variety of disciplines: clergy, physicians, health care agencies and institutions, social workers, concerned humanitarians. The fact that each of these persons could see hospice from the vantage point of his or her own professional perspective meant that, from their founding, hospices were seen as serving a variety of needs. This supported the holistic approach that was very much a part of the prototypical British hospices.

The precipitating factor in becoming a hospice patient is the failure of a healthy body that has been taken for granted for many years. The nature of the illness often produces a great deal of physical pain. The foundations of life are shaken because that which had been trusted is now extremely vulnerable.

But it is apparent that the patient's involvement with physical illness, pain, and approaching death is not exclusively physical. There is social disruption, as the threat of the severing of relations with significant persons is realized, adding the pain of impending separation and of loneliness to physical discomfort.

These losses are accompanied by a threat of loss of meaning. The meanings which enrich our lives are linked to our being. So persons who realize that they are dying pose ultimate questions of meaning. What does death mean? What does *my* death mean? Does my approaching death cut me off from all that has meaning, or can it be integrated into the wholeness that is existence?

Hospice does not limit itself to dealing with the physical illness of the individual, but acknowledges the importance of dealing with the patient and family in all the dimensions of their dying and living. A concerted effort is made to deal holistically with their physical, emotional and spiritual pain.

Theological Implications

Holism is a concept that has often been claimed for Christian theology, but there is a persistent inconsistency in affirming the holistic view. It has been professed that the basic anthropology of the Judeo-Christian tradition is unitary, with the human person seen as a unity of a number of components, usually designated as body, mind, and spirit, held in a tension or balance. But there is also in Christian theology a pronounced strain of confusing dualistic imagery from the Hellenistic tradition: separate realities of physical and spiritual worlds, perishing body and enduring soul. This has made it difficult to affirm unambiguous commitment to the holistic principle.

In spite of the pervasive infusions of Hellenistic dualism, it is possible to understand the Christian theological tradition of becoming whole, or being whole, even in a relative sense, as a normative condition. The tension between relationship and alienation is an important part of theological conceptualization. It is used to describe the interactions between humans and God, between persons, and between elements within a person.

The spiritual dimension can be understood as that force which makes wholeness possible. The concern of the pastor is to enable wholeness, "shalom": to show a way of feeling that one belongs to the center of being, to draw people into more meaningful relationships with their fellow humans, to help persons be in touch with as much as possible of their experience of life—and death. All of these pastoral functions are involved in ministry to hospice patients and families.

Each of the dimensions of human personhood—physical, mental, spiritual—involves a variety of concerns. In the spiritual dimension we have pointed in the prior chapter to the following concerns: belonging and relationship, meaning, self-worth, and coping. Hospice tries to address these concerns and supports a holistic theological anthropology.

The Holistic Context of Hospice

The basic concept behind hospice care is comprehensiveness. It tries to deal with as many dimensions of the patient's life as possible. It involves as many persons as feasible in the care of the patient, representing a broad spectrum of disciplines. It defines care in terms of what the patient wants and needs. A narrow, one-dimensional focus is inimical to the goals of hospice care.

The experience of most hospice patients, prior to their hospice admission, has taken them through a course of investigation, diagnosis, and treatment that has been more and more sharply focused. They have moved from family physician into the care of specialists, whose competence centers on only one part of the patient's being. They have been treated in institutions that also operate on the model of specialized focus. They may be seen by a number of caregivers, whose efforts are understandably specifically and narrowly focused, and who sometimes function without awareness of or appreciation for the efforts of others who are treating the patient.

Once the person becomes involved with hospice, the pattern of care changes abruptly from the specialized to a generalized model. Although caregivers may have specialized competence, they all make a conscious effort to deal with the whole person. Physical pain, family relationships, and a quest for meaning are all intentional concerns of hospice care.

Hospice is shaped by two profound realities: Death is a universal condition (all die), and death is intensely personal (I am dying). The fact that death is part of our common lot does not mean that all people confront death in exactly the same way. The holistic understanding of hospice, which sees persons as complex combinations of a variety of elements, forces the recognition that the needs of patients and families are highly individual and must be met on a personal basis.

Such individual variations exist in all aspects of a person's life. Physical needs, emotional needs, and spiritual needs differ from person to person. A standardized approach, whether medical or psychological or pastoral, is inappropriate.

Hospice experiences a tension between the norms that are implicit in hospice care and the perceptions and experiences of the hospice patient and family. Hospice hopes that people will be accepting of approaching death, but acknowledges that a variety of evasive denials may also be present. Hospice wants to support families in drawing closer together in the crisis of terminality, but knows that some people continue to feel estranged. Hospice intends for people to be aware of the multidimensional nature of their needs and the resources available to deal with them, but sees and understands that some fail to apprehend this complexity.

Hospice cannot and will not reject patients because they are not fully accepting of death, are alienated from one another, or are unaware of the more profound dimensions of existence. But at the same time hospice will continue to function in the light of its normative assumptions: acceptance, relatedness, self-worth, meaning. These attitudes are not forced on people but are quietly modeled as appropriate ways to deal with the crisis of impending death. Whether or not the patient and family act according to that model is their decision.

The organizing center of a hospice program is the impulse to care. Caring is defined as broadly as possible in terms of the needs of the persons, their perceptions of those needs, the interdisciplinary resources hospice can offer, and the attitudes of hospice personnel.

The Person Is the Focus

The focus of hospice on the person has two ramifications. Potentially, hospice has to be prepared to meet a very broad spectrum of needs, because a hospice deals with a great variety of individuals over the course of a year. Actually, hospice has to try its very best to focus on all the unique needs of a particular individual and family.

Wholeness assumes a reasonable inner integrity. When the spiritual dimension is understood as the integrating, unifying element, then to heighten personal integrity is a proper function of spiritual caregiving.

All those who work with hospice are constantly challenged to give full attention to the need of the person, both patient and family, to be himself or herself as fully as possible. Support is given to enable people "to die their own deaths"—to die with integrity, to experience a congruence between the style in which they have lived and in which they now die. Both the dying and those who mourn their deaths are to be able to be themselves. This means that all those who work with hospice have to be fully committed to dealing with individuals in an intensely personalized fashion.

Life Review

Life review is one way of conceptualizing the personal dimension. The place of memory in the grieving process is well known. Mourners are able to sever their emotional ties, to relate to their lost past in new ways, as they participate in an extended process of recollection. Terminally ill persons are also mourners, experiencing anticipatory grief for the life that is drawing to its close. So hospice patients are regularly found in a process of remembering, as they grieve for themselves.

We know how often terminally ill persons find meaning in rehearsing their life experiences. Sometimes this is very tangibly acted out in trips to personally significant places or in reunions with significant people from the past. Sometimes it is overlaid with a reassessment of past actions and relationships. In a sense the dying person is exploring what his or her life has meant, moving toward a synthesis in which the many elements of experience fit together.

A number of pastors who work with hospice patients report that they encounter expressions of guilt rather frequently, guilt which often has a quality of inappropriateness because it is related to long-past events and relationships.

Again this suggests that religion, often through the pastoral relationship, offers an avenue for dealing with the errors and regrets of the past. The Christian practices of confession and forgiveness can be a part of the life-review process. These are ways of affirming that the past does not bind a person inexorably to failure or error or wrongdoing.

> As representatives of a religious community, clergy often serve to remind people of present ties or ones lost in a distant past. In either case the ties are or have been real and function to link us to meanings and persons which help to overcome isolation. Clergy also sometimes symbolize hope to people. They serve to bring to mind the ways in which omissions, defeats, failures, and disappointments may be dealt with and one's life make sense again.[1]

Another way of describing life review is through Glen Davidson's notion of story.[2] Every person develops his or her own life story. We think here not so much of autobiography as of meaning. One's story in some way contains one's picture of meaning: what is real and what is not real, what is known and what is unknown, what is good and what is evil, what is controllable and what is beyond control.

For the dying person, the story takes on new and special meaning. In the normal course of events, we are usually willing to let the story unfold on its own. But a sense of terminality brings an increased desire to shape the ending of the story. This ending may involve some imagining of the way in which the person will face death. It may involve the person's speculation or belief about what follows clinical death.

The human mind, at least in its Western expression, works toward some kind of closure—a completeness, a resolution. As life is terminating, persons have a very understandable concern for completing unfinished business, for righting old wrongs, for drawing together fragments of experience into a meaningful whole, for bringing personal history to its final destination. This need for completion is reflected in a person's story.

While these stories have an intensely personal quality, we also need to recognize that they are shaped by the paradigmatic experiences of family, and the ethnic, religious, and cultural communities of which we are members. We tell our stories with the language and images of the communities that are most influential in our lives.

Those who experience themselves as part of a religious community may express their sense of completeness in religious imagery. Many religious views are focused on a sense of wholeness. Often the belief pattern will deal with the loss of wholeness and its restoration or return, although we need to recognize that sometimes wholeness is achieved by discarding dimensions of the person's existence rather than by trying to integrate them into a unifying whole. Religious ritual often enacts or describes this reorientation to wholeness, whatever form it takes.

As Davidson points out, it is the nature of communities to provide stories that describe how life originated, the destiny toward which it is directed, and how one is to make that journey.[3] Such stories, which are most commonly rooted in the religion of a community, are the guideposts by which individuals orient themselves. They provide a kind of cultural or religious road map by which a person describes his or her course through life. Such a "map" is particularly valuable in times of crisis, when the individual feels somewhat lost or confused. There is real value, then, in helping dying or troubled persons to tell and retell their stories, so that they may be put in touch once again with those symbols that help them know where they are and where they are going.

The pastoral caregiver has some valuable resources

to assist this process. The use of the symbolic language or the symbolic rituals of the persons' religious community in a time of crisis helps people to remember parts of their own stories and encourages the retelling of the story. The recitation of the Twenty-third Psalm or the giving of communion may have a potent and helpful effect on the telling of the personal story of the patient.

One's story is, or ought to be, the manifestation of personal integrity. Hospice believes that one should have the freedom to tell his or her story, including its ending. Those who care for the dying person must have sufficient respect for that freedom, resisting any temptation to detract from the meaningfulness of that story to the person, or to try to reshape the story by imposing their own meanings on it.

It is now recognized that many who worked with the terminally ill in the past decade or so yielded to such temptation. Through a misunderstanding of the structure of the well-known "stages of dying" outlined by Elisabeth Kübler-Ross,[4] the dying person's story was edited by caregivers. Efforts were made to move persons through the structure rather than holding in high regard their freedom to shape their own dying. Such oversimplified understanding of Kübler-Ross seriously compromised the self-determination of the terminally ill and endangered their personal integrity. The personal stories of the dying more often reflect the complexity, the ambiguity, the paradoxical nature of their situations. Part of the person may be accepting of approaching death and another part may be fearful or playing games of denial. The patient's story with its variegated nuance is a much more adequate vehicle for permitting the person to be herself or himself than is patterned theory. Although not so neat, it is a supporter of personal integrity and authenticity.

Two Aspects of Holistic Care

The holistic commitment of hospice is implemented in two major ways: in the style of performance of the individual hospice caregiver and in the inclusion of an interdisciplinary team of caregivers in every hospice organization.

Although one has to be careful not to overly romanticize hospice staff, there is an inevitable existential involvement that supports the holistic approach. Hospice personnel are not incidentally or tangentially involved with dying patients, as may be the case in other health care settings. Hospice staff involvement is highly intentional; these people *choose* to deal with the dying.

The care that they give is not high-tech but high-personal involvement. There is a sharing of the human condition, with all its vulnerability, that bonds many patients and staff members at a profound level. Not only is there deep caring, there is also a common awareness of mortality. In spite of the fact that death is the outcome of every hospice situation, there is in the work of hospice staff the affirmation that compassionate caring and sensitive sharing communicate the possibility of finding meaning in the life that remains.

Hospice functions in our contemporary pluralistic and secularized society, where not all patients and families are deeply rooted in a faith community, nor is every hospice worker necessarily committed to a traditional religious faith. But the holistic approach of hospice makes room for a broad variety of expressions of religious values, not the least of which is that there is more to life than physical health. The interface of finitude and infinity, of isolation and belonging, of resignation and striving, permeates the lives of patients, families, and hospice caregivers.

Professional hospice staff are joined by volunteers who are in no sense medical specialists, but who specialize in caregiving of a personal nature. In keeping with the holistic emphasis of hospice, each worker is implicitly challenged to adopt a broad view of care rather than the narrowly focused approach of the specialist. Growing out of this broad view, experience with a number of hospice staffs has shown that pastoral concerns are brought forward frequently by a wide variety of caregivers.

Holism is manifested also in the formation of an interdisciplinary team in which there are representatives of a number of professions, who bring special competence to caregiving. This team seeks to make certain that all dimensions of the well-being of patient and family are attended to. Physicians and nurses ensure that bodily needs are met. Home health aides, other service personnel, and hospice volunteers pay attention to day-to-day practical needs. Social workers and counselors look to the psychosocial dimensions of care. Pastoral caregivers focus on the spiritual needs of these persons in crisis. Each member of the interdisciplinary team ensures coverage of one of the dimensions of human existence: physical, mental, social, spiritual.

This coverage is done self-consciously with a broad general concern for the whole person: patient or family member. The regularly scheduled meetings allow the interdisciplinary team to communicate about all the needs of the patient and family.

This process of communication within the hospice team is made more valuable by the interdisciplinary nature of the team. The conversations of a number of special competencies around the goal of caring makes clear communication very important. The languages of a number of disciplines must be used to communicate effectively. The peer relationship is a challenge to the impulse for any one discipline to think of itself as the only contributor to the well-being of the patient.

The Pastor as a Member of the Interdisciplinary Team

Parish pastors might relate to the interdisciplinary team in several ways. Many hospices have a pastoral care coordinator or chaplain on their staff, whose responsibility is to facilitate the involvement of the patient's pastor, priest, or rabbi. Or, a pastor whose parishioner becomes a hospice patient can initiate contact with the hospice to coordinate the pastoral care he or she is giving with the services hospice is rendering. Discussions of that patient in the weekly team conference can include the pastor, and contacts can be made between the pastor and hospice workers caring for the patient.

A number of pastors commented on the free exchange that characterized the team's operation. They found that they could often contribute to the team a picture of the patient and family before the onset of the terminal illness, or they could describe the spiritual quest of the patient. They received feedback from the team on where the person was in the dying process and were regularly informed of his or her condition, especially when they were not in daily contact with the patient.

The intentional inclusion of pastors in hospice caregiving programs, for those who wish spiritual care, has often met with success. Some pastors have welcomed the opportunity. One pastor said, "I have the feeling that hospice actually *encourages* pastoral care, while non-hospice health care institutions *permit* it."

The National Hospice Organization Standards, which were adopted in 1979, indicated a desire to include the religious dimension in the work of hospice.

Hospice care is concerned with the dynamic process of religion, that is, with binding together, tying up and tying fast. On the intrapersonal level, hospice endeavors to support the integration of the human personality in the face of the physical deterioration in impending death. The interpersonal dimension of hospice care seeks to promote the development and continuance of significant human relationship(s) between the dying person and other human beings. And finally, in regard to the eschatological dimension of human life, hospice care affirms each person's search for ultimate meaning by respecting and responding to each individual's personal truth.[5]

A revision of these standards stated:

Hospice exists in the hope and belief that, through appropriate care and the promotion of a caring community sensitive to their needs, patients and families may be free to attain a degree of mental and spiritual preparation for death that is satisfactory to them.[6]

As was indicated earlier, both the National Hospice Organization and the Joint Commission on Accreditation of Hospitals, the two major standard-setting organizations for hospices, have stipulated that hospices must serve the spiritual needs of patients and families. They have stated that the clergy should be represented on the interdisciplinary team and have urged regular hospice contact with the religious leadership and spiritual resources of the community.

However, beyond this effort to affirm the holism of the hospice approach, the standards are not explicit in defining spiritual care. Hospices are well aware of the pluralistic religious situation in our culture. Not only is there a broad variety of faith communities in our society, there are many persons who profess no religious commitment. Individual beliefs must be respected, as well as the right to have no specific belief system.

Spiritual care means one thing to a Roman Catholic family, something else to a conservative Protestant family. It is defined yet another way by a Jewish family, still another way by liberal Protestants. Thoroughly secularized persons would have yet another definition. Because hospices have tended to resist a purely sectarian stance and see themselves as community-based organizations, the lack of specific definition is not only understandable, but desirable.

Hospice's intent to focus care on the specific needs of a particular patient and family means that general, broad definitions of spiritual care are abandoned in favor of definitions tailored to the spiritual needs of a particular patient. The pastor who works with hospice has to clarify the difference between this kind of particularity and privatism, in trying to define and meet the spiritual needs of a patient and family. This is not the same thing as insisting that because religious commitment is a private and personal matter, hospice should not be concerned about it. To take the latter stance would deny the holistic assumptions upon which hospice care is based.

Even though it is easy to understand the difficulty of defining spiritual care, this imprecision may cause spiritual concerns to be very peripheral in some hospice care. Pastors working with hospices have to be aware of this danger of marginality, while recognizing also the risks of defining spiritual care in the hospice setting too absolutely and narrowly.

It should be noted that the lack of clarity in defining spiritual care also runs over into the designation of who will provide the care. Joint Commission and NHO standards, as well as current Hospice Medicare requirements, specify that while certain professional members of the interdisciplinary team must be specifically employed by hospices, the functions of the spiritual caregivers may be carried out by non-professionals (employed staff, trained volunteers) or co-opted community clergy.

Although there is general support for having a variety of hospice caregivers be concerned for the spiritual needs of the patient and family, there is also recognition that this is a special form of care. Spiritual caregiving should be at once a shared responsibility of the hospice team and the structured responsibility of one of its professional members, the clergyperson.

For a great many people it is quite natural to involve the clergy in situations of severe crisis. There is a kind of ultimacy in their situations that calls them to ask serious questions. They want someone who can talk with them about the meaning of living and dying, someone who is committed to caring. But for the person who does not want it, or who does not want it *now*, hospice does not impose pastoral care. The pastor's commitment to the right of the patient to privacy or solitude prevents forcing a visit on the person. Initiative is limited to informing the patient that a pastoral resource is available through hospice on request.

Some hospices have the impression that a few pastors are happy to have hospice step in because it relieves them of major responsibility. Other hospices point to difficulties they have had involving pastors, particularly in visits to non-church families who have asked for a pastoral visit. They have found pastors who resist "making house calls," and others who are unwilling to face death in the open way which hospice affirms. This may be due to personal anxieties about death or to a kind of Pollyanna theology which prefers sweetness and light to the harsher realities of life and death. In such situations hospice may be a painful, but constructive, reminder to pastors that adequate ministry meets people where they are.

There are a number of activities involving patients and families that are proper functions of the pastoral caregiver as a member of the hospice team. These include helping persons understand and articulate their spiritual needs; exploring those things which they value ultimately; talking about their understandings of death and its consequences; offering sacraments, rituals, and funerals; and maintaining the relationship of the family in crisis to the ongoing life of the faith community.

Role Clarification

Before hospice, in modern times most deaths occurred in hospitals or similar settings. One pastor said, "I used to dread going to a dying person, largely because I didn't know what I could do." He was saying that he had no sense of what his pastoral role might be. Hospice can make a difference by helping pastors to a new understanding of what they can provide for dying persons and their families.

In the strongly authoritarian hospital setting, pastors have often found themselves very unsure of their place. They have been intimidated, by the exotic interventions of medical technology, into feeling that they had very little help to offer. They have felt that they have been in an adversarial relationship with the authoritarian structure of the modern medical center, struggling for earlier entrée for their pastoral caregiving than at the terminus of treatment: "Call the pastor; there is nothing more we can do."

Pastoral identity is not easy to establish in such a setting. The technologies of scientific medicine are so impressive and spiritual caregiving so poorly defined that pastoral functions are easily consigned to irrelevant gentility.

One pastor said, "In hospice people see me as a friend, so there is no great difference between lay and professional caregivers. In the hospital I am more role conscious because I feel I have to justify my presence in a setting with a strong professional hierarchy."

It is not difficult to see why pastors would find clarification for their pastoral role in hospice. In that setting, caregiving involves support, empathy, love, and acceptance. These are the traditional components of ministry. As one pastor said, "Hospice is a natural extension of what my ministry is all about." The hospice setting is different from the hospital in two ways. First, here medical high technology is irrelevant; simple caring is the chief mode of treatment. Second, there is a commitment to the holistic approach in a non-hierarchical structure in which every hospice caregiver is to be concerned for the whole person of the patient. Families see the clergy as an ally and a *direct caregiver* for themselves as well as for the patient. Knowing that the pastor is part of the team that touches their lives in so many ways helps to build the pastoral relationship.

Summary

In hospice the holistic approach is both theoretically and practically followed. Efforts are made to be responsive to a variety of dimensions of the experience of the patient: physical, emotional, and spiritual, and the perspectives and competencies of a variety of interdisciplinary resources are offered. Because caring is at the center of this approach, the pastor has a meaningful role in this process.

NOTES

1. Liston O. Mills, "Issues for Clergy in the Care of the Dying and Bereaved," in *Dying and Death*, ed. David Burton (Baltimore: Williams & Wilkins, 1977), p. 201.

2. Glen W. Davidson, *The Hospice: Development and Administration*, 2nd ed. (Washington: Hemisphere Publishing Corp., 1985), pp. 171ff.

3. Ibid., p. 146.

4. Elisabeth Kübler-Ross, *On Death and Dying* (New York: Macmillan, 1969).

5. National Hospice Organization, *Standards of a Hospice Program of Care* (Arlington, Va.: National Hospice Organization, 1979).

6. National Hospice Organization, *Standards of a Hospice Program of Care* (Arlington, Va.: National Hospice Organization, 1982).

CHAPTER 3

OPENNESS IN DEALING WITH DEATH

People have to ask to be admitted to a hospice program. Although referrals may come from physicians, hospitals, clergy, friends, or family, the process of admission involves an assessment visit in which the hospice concept and program is carefully explained to the patient and his or her family. Only then do the patient and family decide whether or not to enter the hospice program.

In a sense, then, hospice requires a measure of "acceptance" of approaching death as a condition of admission. The decision to become a hospice patient usually symbolizes the giving up of hope for a cure and the acknowledgment that palliative treatment is the only available option. It is not unusual for patients and families to take some time to make this decision, unless circumstances of caring for the patient lend urgency.

Experience shows that there are those rare instances in which a person who has been diagnosed as terminal recovers or goes into extended remission. Such reversals of the course of the disease are relatively infrequent in hospice programs because most people do not enter programs until the prognosis is a few months or less. Some may exceed the remaining time predicted, but only very rarely does a person recover sufficiently to be released from the program.

Entering a hospice program represents a very significant and complicated transition. It means careful assessment of the future; it involves definition of one's most precious hopes; it requires a reshaping of attitudes and behaviors. In many instances it means that members of the family will be taking on sizable and, often, unfamiliar home-care responsibilities.

As we shall see shortly in more detail, there is a measure of acceptance of approaching death involved, although some denial systems may well continue to operate. Patients and families rarely are completely accepting of death. It is much more common to find patients shuttling between acceptance and denial. Part of the effective functioning of hospice is to provide a level of caring (physically, emotionally, spiritually) that will support the patient and family enough for a sizable measure of acceptance to be achieved. Hospice does not court the acceptance of terminality, but neither does it shy away from that acceptance when time seems to dictate it. Hospice deals with approaching death openly in a context of caring.

The openness fostered by hospice participation is obviously helpful to patients and families. Game playing is not needed. The "double charade" of both patient and family pretending that the patient is not terminally ill is no longer necessary. Many patients who are aware of the seriousness of their illness want to make the most of the time remaining for them. They realize how precious are opportunities to talk with those who are most important to them. And many families find themselves able to express their perceptions and feelings more honestly. Openness fosters a level of communication that offers the possibility for deepening relationship in this time of crisis.

How Hospice Helps to Achieve Openness

Hospice has a rather sharply focused agenda: enabling the patient to live the remaining days to the fullest, relieving pain, fostering relationships, and opening communication. This contrasts with the more complicated agenda that existed before admission to hospice. That agenda included a variety of possible treatments for the illness, hope for total or partial recovery, and a more nebulous prognosis. The patient felt many more options were open. Then, the progress of the disease and the lack of successful treatment reduced the number of options. Admission to hospice involves a far less ambiguous course, fostering openness and a clarity about the immediate future that resists subterfuge.

Hospice staff help by modeling openness in their dealings with patients and families. This does not mean cruel frankness, but it does involve real honesty and unwillingness to play games. The very presence of hospice is a silent reminder of the real situation. Open conversations with hospice staff describe honestly the patient's situation and deal candidly with the patient's concerns. This establishes a pattern for open communication between patients and families.

The language that is used in the hospice situation is crucial in establishing openness. Familiar euphemisms are not used, but accurate non-technical terminology is employed when discussing the patient's condition. People know that a great effort is being made to be honest. Issues are not avoided but are dealt with openly in the context of caring and support. Family members are encouraged to ask their questions and to expect honest answers.

Hospice staff members are specifically trained to deal with death. They have developed sufficient understanding of their own mortality, so that they do not have to be defensive in their vulnerability. They can communicate comfortably with patients and families about death. They are less tempted to engage in the conventional diversions from discussions of death. This sets a tone that is very liberating to hospice families, who express their appreciation again and again for being able to share openly and honestly in the process of living until death happens.

The Effect of Openness on Pastoral Care

It is debatable whether difficulty in accepting death is part of the existential human situation or a distinctive component of Western cultural attitudes toward death. Instinctive self-preservation is sometimes interpreted as an indicator of the foreign, intrusive nature of death in human experience. This would suggest to some that denial and rebellion are more appropriate human responses, at least in Western culture, than acceptance.

One does not have to make an absolute choice between acceptance and denial. It is more helpful to think of this in terms of an ongoing struggle. The pastoral task, then, is to join people where they are in their struggle and to help them by talking about the tension they feel between acceptance and denial. There is no need to "push" acceptance or to collapse denial. The simple process of talking about both of these dimensions is helpful to the movement of the patient and family toward greater acceptance.

In some health care systems, patients and their families receive no specific encouragement to deal openly with their situations. They are not given full particulars of their condition. They are urged to be less than candid with one another in discussing the prognosis. Many pastors are familiar with situations in which well-intentioned people try to protect one another from facing the fact of approaching death. In one family the patient and her husband were reasonably accepting, but their parents were insistent that the patient was "looking better." They urged the patient, against her wishes, to go from one specialist to another in hope of finding a cure, all without success. These members of the family could not face the fact that death was nearing, even when it was only days away. The pastor and hospice workers did not argue with these parents but reflected how difficult and painful it was for them to think about their daughter's illness. The patient and her husband were supported when they offered their perceptions of the situation.

The pastor is faced with the same task as the family, namely, letting go, being willing to give up the patient. One pastor commented, "I draw the conclusion, from behavior of some local clergy serving their parishioners, that some pastors have a hard time letting go, and thus may be less apt to be open." Openness may challenge the helper's denial responses. The pastor, like any member of the hospice staff, needs to recognize that he or she also participates in this struggle of acceptance and denial. The openness of hospice makes such acknowledgment possible, as well as providing a means for dealing with it.

Hospice tries to make a difference by being open, and is often successful. One pastor said, "In hospice I usually do not fear that some people are trying to hide the fact of oncoming death from the patient." Another reported, "In hospice I am not the only one to broach the subject of death." This suggests that in non-hospice settings pastors have felt very unsure about just how directly they should be approaching the dying patient. In hospice, however, the pastor can be assured that the entire program is functioning with openness. The reality of approaching death is not a taboo subject, nor are devious intrigues required. This produces a context in which both pastor and patient can be comfortable in their discussions of approaching death. As one pastor put it, "People 'name their demons' more readily in hospice programs."

It is easy for partisans of hospice to idealize or oversimplify the effects of hospice involvement. One might assume that all hospice patients and families are fully accepting of the death that is coming closer, that all conversations are rich with meaning, that all attitudes are composed and positive. However, in spite of thoughtful openness, some patients or family members are not able to hear what is being said.

Openness should not be taken to be synonymous with acceptance of death. As stated earlier, most people tend to experience tension between acceptance and denial. This manifests itself in several possible ways. Sometimes there is alternation of periods of acceptance and denial; sometimes it involves rational acceptance and emotional denial.

This ambivalence was effectively illustrated by a terminally ill pastor who discussed his situation with a seminary class. He was a model of "terminal candor," having faced his death with genuine openness in his own family and in the community. However, he chose to talk to the seminarians about all the ways in which he also acted out denial of his death, acknowledging that even his willingness to talk about his approaching death was a way of reminding himself that it hadn't happened yet.

Many people understood the familiar "five stages of dying" of Elisabeth Kübler-Ross to mean that one moved from denial to acceptance in a fixed pattern of escalation.[1] Dealing with many hospice patients shows that even persons who are quite accepting of their deaths have some denial systems operating. Acceptance, then, is relative, on a personal basis. Because hospice is dedicated to dealing with people where they are, it will not press upon them a stance that is not really theirs. If people want to deny approaching death, that is their right. Hospice will not overtly support their denial, nor will hospice deliberately destroy it. Not only is it hoped that patients and families will be open in their approach to death; hospice must also be open in permitting people to be themselves in their stances toward dying.

So too with pastoral care. It is not the goal of the pastor to compel people to be fully accepting of death, even though that is the attitude we might wish for them. The pastoral caregiver, in step with hospice staff, supports the level of acceptance that obtains for the patient and family and does not argue with the denial that is present. Openness is the more appropriate goal.

The openness of the hospice setting makes such pastoral conversation much easier. The fundamental assumption in the hospice philosophy of the right of the patient to be himself or herself promotes a fertile environment for the pastor to let people talk about the way in which their accrued life experiences, their attitudes, their faith commitment or its absence, are involved in their grappling with the tension between acceptance and denial.

In the very late stages of this struggle there is often, but not necessarily, a tipping of the scales toward acceptance. This may be accompanied by a kind of disengagement, a letting go, a detachment from relationships, a movement into solitude. One patient, whose family would not give up in the search for heroic treatment, insisted that there was no need for further struggle. Formerly a loquacious person, she became increasingly quiet. She slept or feigned sleep a good deal. She frequently talked with the hospice nurse about her wish for the end to come.

For religiously oriented people, this movement may be conceptualized in the imagery of their faith as a transition from the present life to new life, however that may be understood. Munley observes:

The social environment in which death occurs is clearly a world of feeling as well as of meaning. A striking feature of the hospice context is that patients are usually able to bring their struggle between resisting and yielding to a close in a way that harmonizes with individual personalities and total life experiences. Repeatedly I witnessed the tranquility of religiously oriented patients whose conflict between hanging on and letting go of life ended in a yielding to that which they considered "divine."[2]

Summary

In the midst of a society that has only recently begun to move from a death-denying stance toward an affirmation that death is a part of life, the pastor joins parishioners in the struggle to accept as fully as possible approaching death. The candor which hospice tries to bring to the situation offers support for the exploration of the deepest feelings about death of all those who find themselves in a situation of terminality.

NOTES

1. Elisabeth Kübler-Ross, *On Death and Dying* (New York: Macmillan, 1969).

2. Anne Munley, *The Hospice Alternative* (New York: Basic Books, 1983), p. 231f.

CHAPTER 4

PAIN CONTROL AND THE PASTOR

Hospice has focused particular attention on pain control, recognizing that ever increasing pain is an issue for many of its patients. Not only have new pain-relieving medications been developed, but new attitudes and procedures for the administration of such medications have been advanced.

Much has been learned about the physiology and psychology of patients who experience extreme pain. Pain control has become a medical specialty, and a number of centers that specialize in the treatment of chronic and severe pain have opened. The terminality of the hospice patient sets that dimension of pain control off from the rest of the pain control field. Treatment of a person with chronic lower back pain or advanced arthritis is quite different from that of the person with cancer whose life expectancy, according to best knowledge, is measured in weeks.

Most hospice patients suffer from cancer. Some forms of this disease are more painful than others. The location of the primary malignancy and the points of the body to which it has metastasized provide the hospice staff with preliminary information about the kinds of pain that can be anticipated. Because the disease is progressive, it can be expected in many cases that the experience of pain will also be progressive. It is, therefore, quite likely that pain medication will have to be changed frequently to deal with increasing pain. Relief from pain is temporary, requiring that some way be found to spare the patient the anguish of returning discomfort.

In many illnesses, pain is part of the healing process. In the postoperative patient, there is pain from the illness being treated and pain produced as an aftermath of the surgical procedure. Not only is this pain temporary, expected to last only a few days in severe form, it is also clearly associated with the recovery of the patient. It is easier to accept the pain in the expectation that "things have to get worse before they can get better."

Chronic pain presents a somewhat different picture. This is usually pain that has not yielded easily to treatment. It is often associated with illnesses that are not life-threatening, such as problems in the spine or other bones or migraine headaches. The pain is severe, protracted, and difficult to relieve, and treatment for the pain must take into account that life will go on for the patient.

But the hospice patient is dying. This affects the situation in two ways. First, there is the addition of physical pain to the emotional pain of recognizing that life is drawing to a close and that separation from loved ones will occur. Second, it is death, not renewed health, that will provide relief. Pain will not go on, in most instances, for seemingly endless time.

Because pain is experienced by the majority of hospice patients, prime attention is given to treating it. Not only is this approach based upon very basic humane impulses, but it also recognizes that unless pain is relieved, it totally preoccupies the patient, limiting the other supportive measures that can be helpful to the dying patient. One of the first tasks hospice addresses when a person is admitted to the program is the effective control of pain.

Hospice care approaches pain control by providing the best medical treatment available for it. It also recognizes the psychological, social, and spiritual dimensions of pain and its treatment. This awareness guides the activities of the members on the interdisciplinary team in collaboratively addressing the pain control needs of the patient. The dosage of pain-relieving medication, the loving support of family members, the positioning of the patient in bed by the nurse, the social worker's dealing with economic needs of the family, the volunteer's willingness to sit with the patient for hours, the pastor's openness to listening to the patient reach out for possible meaning in his or her approaching death—in all of these ways hospice is working on pain control.

Hospice understands that if any of these areas of the patient's experience are not touched, pain control will not be fully effective. It also recognizes that unless these dimensions of pain are controlled, the goal of helping the person to live as fully as possible in his or her remaining time is not met.

Pastoral Care and Pain Control

As part of the interdisciplinary team, the pastor plays a role in pain control. He or she shares the concern for all dimensions of pain control with other members of the team but can make a distinctive contribution to its relief.

Because the fundamental stance of the biblical tradition is to deal with life rather than to try to evade it, pain and suffering are frequently encountered. Metaphors of childbirth, stories of slavery, persecution, and warfare, and accounts of martyrdom culminate in a paradigmatic crucifixion. Pain is ended as part of human experience only in eschatological visions.

Like many dimensions of the human situation seen from the spiritual perspective of Christian tradition, the nature of pain is described paradoxically. On the one hand, pain is interpreted as punishment or judgment; on the other, suffering is seen as redemptive. Pain is associated with those experiences in which persons and peoples feel cut off or abandoned by God. In other instances pain is the occasion for affirming that God is nearest when suffering is most severe. The ultimate understanding of the compassionate God sees God sharing in the suffering of humanity and of an individual person.

It is probably fair to say that pastors encounter the negative side of this paradox more frequently. Pastors interviewed described hospice patients who ask, "What have I done to deserve this?" or "I guess I am being punished for smoking all those years," or "Why am I being punished? I've always tried to do my best."

While some such views directly relate personal behavior to punishment through pain, contemporary understandings of the way the environment has been polluted, knowingly or unknowingly, with carcinogens, causing widespread cancers, dilute this understanding. The punishment motif is not credible when it is discovered that a commonly acceptable food or behavior contributes to the onset of a life-threatening disease.

Similarly, the awareness in our time that, for example, particular industries endanger public health by dumping industrial wastes or by spreading radioactivity makes the thought of the individual being punished by his or her disease less relevant. In fact, it has been suggested that the increasing practice of suing those deemed liable for the circumstances which caused a death has become the way of dealing with the guilt and anger frequently involved in mourning. Finding a target for responsibility, even legitimate responsibility, outside oneself removes guilt and the sense of being punished. Rather, one becomes an agent for punishing the external cause of the death, through litigation.

However, there still are many times that a pastor encounters the inference that pain is personal punishment, in the seriously ill. This ancient feeling goes far back into the roots of human experience to a primitive, pre-logical way of understanding life.

Attitudes Toward Pain

In their very helpful book, *People in Pain: Guidelines for Pastoral Care*, Wayne and Charles Oates describe four kinds of attitudes toward pain: denial, stoicism, magical thinking, and realism.[1]

Denial is produced by social or religious pressures that convince the person that he or she ought not to give in to admitting pain. The "big boys don't cry" conditioning is not limited strictly to males. There is a general disposition in much of Western culture to hold back on expressions of pain, and by implication on having pain. Stiff-upper-lip restraint or the pious affirmation that faith should spare one from suffering are denial postures. Some assume, "If only my faith is strong enough, my pain will go away." Sometimes the denial is intrapersonal; the person is able to condition himself or herself to the view that the pain does not or should not exist, or that physical experiences should be fully subordinated to more worthy spiritual impulses.

A stoical attitude is a kind of acceptance of pain as one's fate. The vernacular phrase "That's the way the cookie crumbles" (or the more sophisticated "c'est la vie") and the religious phrase "It's God's will" are typical expressions of stoical submission to the way things are. Such expressions are fairly common in contemporary experience, but more often they are clichés that express a superficial attitude. This kind of passive submission is manifested far less frequently in persons' behavior.

Magical thinking, the third kind of approach, has a primitive, childish overtone; it is a variant of what Freud called "infantile omnipotence." A non-rational linkage of wish and fact assumes that a person is very special and can control his or her reality. Pastors sometimes encounter people in desperate situations who are seeking some way out of their pain through a one-time divine intervention in the natural order. One hospice patient, upon being told by his physician and family that chemotherapy was being counterproductive, began to insist that Jesus was shrinking the large mass in his abdomen.

Realism in one sense follows the approach we have described as stoicism—acknowledging and accepting that pain is a natural part of the human condition of finiteness and frailty. It is the way we are. But realism goes beyond stoicism to a more active utilization of suffering. This is not simple heroics but the recognition that human beings can relate to their situations, even when desperate, in creative ways. The situations themselves may not change as much as the way in which persons relate to their circumstances.

Pain has a variety of meanings, according to the different interpretations of individuals. For example, the description of pain by the patient is a symptom used by the physician in making a diagnosis. The location, severity, timing, and nature of the pain are important data in giving the pain medical meaning. This diagnosis enables the physician to prescribe treatment for the pain and, when possible, for the underlying condition.

Pain has meaning for those who are around the sufferer. Very often behavior that indicates that the patient is experiencing pain will stimulate compassionate behavior by those who care for the patient. Such responses to the pain of another person range all the way from administering pain-relieving medication to supportive hand holding. The expression of pain is interpreted as a cry for help.

For the pain-bearer pain has a private meaning. Whether it is interpreted as punishment or as an occasion for growth, somehow the patient seeks a meaning in pain. Several levels of approach are functioning, probably simultaneously. Some of the meaning may be non-rational and pre-logical. Some may be cognitive and rational. The language and imagery of one's religious or philosophical commitment are used in an effort to put the pain into a larger perspective. Meaningless pain is the most intolerable, so it is understandable that patients will try to see some purpose behind their suffering. It is not simply the physical sensation but the larger picture that is involved.

The Essentially Personal Nature of Pain

Only a very limited part of the experience of pain can be shared with other persons. The physical experience, of course, is limited to the person who has it. It is simply non-transferable. Accepting the patient's report that he or she has pain, therefore, requires a relationship of trust. Family members, caregivers, and the pastor need sufficient trust in the patient to accept as a fact that the person has pain. That trust needs to be communicated as sensitive awareness that the pain is real indeed to the patient. Compassionate response to the expression of pain is a token of that trust, helping to break down the terrible isolation produced by the loneliness of having a difficult experience that cannot be shared.

The interpretations which the person gives of the sensation are only partially communicable. Because we are conditioned to communicate through rational discourse, rational interpretations of the pain are shared with greatest ease. The non-rational, feeling-level meanings which the person finds are much more difficult to share.

Because some means for sharing is one of the great needs of the patient with pain, caregivers must make a serious effort to take seriously both the fact that the person is experiencing pain and the meanings which the patient has given to the pain. One need not necessarily agree with the meanings, but one has to begin by accepting where the patient is. To start by arguing with the interpretations given to the pain by the patient only increases the sense of isolation.

Caregivers must be aware not only of the difficulties in communicating pain, because of its essentially private nature, but also that some people have difficulty in communicating anything. Verbal communication about pain depends on a patient's capacity for introspection, on the symbol system available to the person, and on the ability to articulate. It is not a coincidence that we refer to stoical persons as "the strong, silent type." The basic stance of passive resignation requires the least interpretation.

It is here that family members and pastors, who have had an extended relationship with the patient, can be helpful to other members of the caregiving team who have been associated with the patient only during this illness. The patient's normal capacity for verbal communication is an important datum in developing sensitive awareness of the patient's pain on the part of all caregivers.

There is also a non-verbal dimension of this communication. Restlessness, wincing, groans, sudden intake of breath, and grimaces are all ways in which the fact of pain is communicated non-verbally. Most such behaviors are largely involuntary, spontaneous products of the physical sensations of pain. Caregivers must be as responsive to these clues as to verbal communication.

A deep existential loneliness is created by the radical way in which one's system of meaning—religious faith, philosophy of life, value structure—is threatened by the onset of extreme pain. Most of our lifetime is relatively pain-free. Most of us do not live with a sense of terrible limitation. We tend to deal with our human frailty and vulnerability largely in the abstract. When pain makes this frailty very concrete, our spiritual resources are severely strained, even to the breaking point. We feel cut off from everything: "My God, my God, why have you forsaken me!"

The only potentially helpful response to such isolation is for another, or others, to *be there for the patient*. True caregiving, especially pastoral caregiving, involves presence. One stands by the patient doggedly, refusing to be frightened away by the fact of the pain or the difficulty the patient is experiencing in sharing it. Theologically stated, the disruption of the cycle of dereliction is by the breaking through of grace. Pastorally, the sense of terrifying isolation is dispelled by the caring presence of others, in spite of the fact that pain cannot be truly shared.

However, having said this, we must recognize the need for pastoral sensitivity to the patient's signals that he or she wishes to be alone part of the time, even with pain. The patient may not necessarily want the pastor's visit at this time, or may not want a visit from the pastor at all. Even though a pastor may have sincere concern for the patient, it is not good pastoral care to impose one's presence.

The emphasis of hospice on individualized care of patients is extremely relevant at this point. The focus on relationship with the patient, the provision of care in familiar, comfortable settings when possible, the participatory process of decision making, all facilitate patients' communication with caregivers about their pain. The understanding that caregivers achieve will be imperfect, but sufficient to permit them to care for patients in ways that relieve their terrible loneliness.

Understanding Pain Medically and Psychologically

Oates and Oates provide a very helpful physiological and psychological understanding of pain, which is important for all caregivers to know. They base their approach on the conceptualization of pain of William Fordyce, differentiating pain from pain behavior.[2] Pain develops from the stimulus of heat or pressure on nerve endings; the resulting electrochemical reaction in the nervous system is experienced as pain. This physical reaction produces an emotional response, suffering, which occurs as the higher centers of the nervous system reflect on the pain. Suffering, in turn, initiates pain behavior: crying out, groaning, grimacing, seeking help, and withdrawing from activity. The movement is from physical event through emotional response to the mobilization of behavior that reflects the discomfort that the body is experiencing. This distinction between pain and pain behaviors is extremely important for caregivers because while pain is not apparent to the observer, pain behavior is. It becomes the medium of communication of the pain from one person to another.

Pain behavior, as Oates and Oates indicate, is made up both of simple reflex actions—wincing, gasping, writhing—and learned behavior, such as calling the attention of caregivers to the pain, talking about the pain, lethargy, social withdrawal, and requesting or taking medication.[3]

Because pain is an experience full of dread, it is understandable that it produces anxiety. The patient with pain is anxious about many elements of that experience. Will the pain get more severe? Can the pain be relieved? Even if relieved, how soon will it return? These are perfectly natural concerns and must be recognized by the caregivers.

Anxiety in the hospice patient is not restricted to concern about pain. There is an even more potent anxiety related to approaching death and its consequences, to separation from loved ones and its effect on them. These all link together to produce a highly stressful situation. Stress, if not dealt with, pyramids, increasing pain behaviors which intensify the pain itself.

It is almost folk wisdom to say that the anticipation of pain is as bad as the pain itself. We know that the dread of something may create so much stress that it accentuates the pain. This kind of psychological pressure is often handled effectively by talking about it.

Anxiety is associated with things that are perceived to be out of control. This creates a profound helplessness in the patient and family. They feel swept into a maelstrom that will suck them down to an even worse situation than the present one, unless some way can be found to enable them to regain a measure of the control they have lost.

Pain can be totally preoccupying. When severe pain, both physical and psychic, is present, the circumference of life is drawn in; attention cannot be given to new experiences or to deeper reflection on present experience. This is felt as a deprivation, since we are accustomed to the excitement and joy of an expanding world of experience.

This constriction of one's world by pain also affects relationships with others. Because, as already said, pain is a very private experience, it stands as a potent reminder that in some things we stand alone. Pain behaviors cannot remove the loneliness completely.

We know from the work of Harry Stack Sullivan and others that stress and anxiety are contagious. When these are experienced by one person in a relationship, they are easily passed on to others. Although only the hospice patient is experiencing the physical pain of the disease, it affects all of those around. Sometimes its effect is to call out empathy and compassion from family and caregivers, drawing people more closely together. Sometimes it overloads the circuits of relationships and produces more stress, even impatience or anger. This can set up a cycle of guilt, which adds to the stress. Or the patient's behavior may become highly manipulative, in an effort to regain some control, causing estrangement in a time when closeness is most needed.

Hospice Treatment of Pain

The overall nature of hospice treatment of pain is based on the concept of control, in response to the feelings of helplessness encountered by the patient and family. They feel that their lives have totally gotten out of control: Nothing can be done.

Hospice is intent upon demonstrating in living experience that we never exhaust the possibilities for doing something. With medication, with quality caregiver support, with open communication, with strengthened family relationships, many of the sources of the patient's and the family's pain can be addressed.

One of the great contributions of the hospice movement has been the recognition that the pain of the patient in late-stage terminal illness must be dealt with differently than the pain of other types of patients.

According to Oates and Oates, as well as reports of many experiences with terminally ill patients, physicians commonly undertreat pain.[4] The situation is described by Oates and Oates:

> Fear of addiction keeps many pain patients from taking minimum amounts even of non-addictive

medications. Some patients have a stoical attitude about pain and think they should be able to "take it." Others, such as the cancer patients studied by John Bonica of the University of Washington, are often undermedicated because of the reluctance of physicians to prescribe enough medication for them.[5]

The protocols worked out to prevent overdependence on narcotics are based on administering as little analgesic medication as possible. This is a reasonable and justifiable policy for the majority of patients. But it is an inappropriate response in many situations of extreme pain in late stage terminal illness.

The pattern of administration of pain-controlling medicines has also been affected by the same policy. The strategy was to wait for the return of pain before administering the next dose of the medication. This is the familiar "p.r.n." ("as needed") regimen, in which medication is not administered until the patient demonstrates a need for it. This means that pain must be experienced again and again to obtain relief. In a situation where the protocol is designed to prevent drug dependence through minimal administration, this may be a valid approach, but its relevance in late-stage terminal illness is questionable.

Because of the serious problem of drug abuse in our society, it is understandable that careful attention is given to measures that might lead to addiction. Medical treatment procedures need to reflect that concern when it is appropriate. But addiction is an irrelevant concern for a person whose remaining life is measured in weeks or days. There is no intelligent trade-off between extreme unrelieved pain and drug dependency when life is radically time-limited.

So deep is the concern for addiction in our society that hospice patients and their families, as well as some physicians, are not able to differentiate between the situation of late-stage terminality and other painful illnesses. Sometimes patients or families will not give the prescribed dosage or follow the schedule for administration, because they do not want the patient to be addicted.

Another concern frequently voiced by hospice patients and families is their desire to maintain lucidity and avoid extended stuporous states. It is not uncommon for the terminally ill to feel that they are caught in a current that is sweeping them toward death, and they feel powerless. This is why it is so important for them to remain conscious and lucid rather than stuporous.

Hospice, with its heavy emphasis on the value of personal interaction between the patient and others, supports this concern and is able, in the majority of cases, to give the kind and dosage of medication that will not keep the patient "snowed under" for extended periods. However, one hospice reported that a patient regularly took only half of the prescribed medication, even though he continued to experience some pain. Visits from family and friends were extremely important to this patient, and he wanted to be alert and able to converse. In spite of assurances from hospice caregivers that if the prescribed dosages were given on the scheduled care plan, the patient would be both lucid and pain-free, the half doses still were taken. The goals of hospice include both pain control and fostering communication between a patient and his or her family and friends.

When medication is administered to relieve pain in a seriously ill person, the relief is temporary and a cyclical pattern is established: pain—medication—relief—return of pain. Under such a regimen the relief is often brief because even before the pain itself returns, the patient is becoming increasingly anxious in anticipation of the return of the pain.

We have already pointed to the standard non-hospice approach of administering medications when the patient demonstrates a need. This is further complicated in routine medical procedures by prescribing a minimum time between dosages to prevent administration in response to the anticipation of pain rather than the pain itself. This is justifiable when there is a valid interest in undermedicating to prevent drug dependence.

Sometimes a patient's or a family's concern grows out of the pragmatic assumption that if a narcotic is used now, it will lose its effectiveness as the pain gets worse. So people hold back lest they reach the time when the medication will be ineffective. Usually the hospice staff can explain that a variety of medications are available and that large doses can be administered without losing effectiveness.

Hospice care makes a concerted effort to regulate the dosages and the schedule for administration to the needs of a particular patient, rather than applying standardized routines. Medication is given shortly before the pain recurs. Once the patient experiences being pain-free and is aware that medications are being planned specifically for his or her situation, the anxiety of anticipating the return of severe pain diminishes and pain is further reduced. The recently developed technique of using small pumps to automatically release frequent, very small doses of medication directly into the bloodstream can be effective for many hospice patients. For many others pain-controlling narcotics are administered by mouth, so that family members do not have to give them by injection.

For some patients additional medication that lowers their anxiety levels can be an important element in controlling their pain. This is particularly helpful for persons with a low threshold for pain or with the background of a long, very painful illness.

Equally important in pain control is the quality of caring that is given. The holistic commitment of hospice makes a caring response, such as "What is it you want?" as important as effective medication. The kinds of medications used and the individualized patterns for administration contribute to the message that the quality of the person's life is of utmost importance.

The hospice team, including the pastor, models an empathic approach that takes the pain of the person very seriously and utilizes every therapeutic modality in its treatment. Although the administration of analgesics is extremely important, it is by no means the whole response of hospice to the pain of the patient. Caring for the emotional and spiritual elements of the patient's and the family's pain is equally central. For example, the visit of a hospice nurse is not simply a matter of giving a medication to the patient, repositioning him or her in bed, and then leaving. The visit will also involve some unhurried conversation with the patient, sometimes in connection with giving a bath and other personal care, but often in just sitting down for a chat. Often, but not necessarily, this can grow into a very important discussion of some concerns that are very much on the mind of the patient or family member. Certainly the call of the pastor can involve much the same.

The relationship between supportive caring and the relief of physical pain is explained by what is called the "placebo effect." Many studies have demonstrated that pain can often be relieved by a placebo, a substance which appears to be the medicine but which has no medicinal effect on the pain. The efficacy of placebos has been explained both psychologically and biochemically. It can be shown that the placebo effect is a symbol of the patient's trust in the ability of the doctor to help. But it can also be shown that the reduction of anxiety achieved through administration of a placebo increases the levels of endorphins, proteins in the brain which participate in relieving pain in much the same way as morphine. Putting these two findings together, researchers conclude that the fact that patients expect help may actually assist them in creating their own biochemical pain relief. So placebos do not simply play tricks on patients; they have a genuine pharmacologic effect.

The Role of Pastoral Care in Pain Control

Pain control relates to pastoral care in two ways. On one hand, uncontrolled pain can preoccupy a patient so much that pastoral ministry is very difficult. On the other hand, pastoral care is one of the ways in which some measure of pain control can be secured. These two facts do not necessarily cancel each other out, but they do produce a tension that inhibits full pastoral effectiveness.

The pastor assists in pain relief by addressing stresses that exacerbate physical pain: the anxiety of the patient, interpersonal tensions, his or her struggles toward meaning. These are not neutral elements in the situation but are actual factors in the pain. Dealing with them effectively can contribute to an easing of the pain, certainly by reducing the well known psychological components of the pain experience and perhaps even biochemically through the placebo effect created by the patient's anticipation of help.

Wayne Oates describes this ministry:

> Herein, then, is the crux of the pastoral care of pain patients: that we suspend our own judgments about the validity or lack of validity of their perception of pain; that we respond to their cry for help by entering *their* world as they perceive it; that we join with them in seeking and collecting all data that can be known about the sources and nature of their pain; that we build a life support community around them to help in bearing and modifying their pain; that the fellowship of learning itself will change beneficially both their perception of pain and the pain itself; and that we do all these things as servants of Jesus Christ and in his name.[6]

77

Hospice management of pain is a good example of the reciprocity between pastoral care and the ministrations of the other members of the interdisciplinary team. Just as the pain-relieving treatment of the physician and nurse help to open the way for effective pastoral relationship, the pastor can support their treatment by helping to reduce the patient's anxiety, by supporting the prescribed use of drugs for those who are reluctant to take them, by joining patients in their search to find meaning in their situation.

Some pastors interviewed for this book described ways in which they had ministered to parishioners who were in pain (although most indicated that such assistance was not a major part of their pastoral care of hospice patients, once pain control had been established). One told how he read and talked briefly about Psalm 13, a psalm of lament, giving the person, as it were, permission to voice her protests to God. Another spoke of simply sitting at the bedside of a parishioner and offering quieting prayer during periods of pain. A Roman Catholic priest described a conversation about Jesus on the cross, after which the patient conceptualized her experience as offering her suffering to God in Jesus' example.

In addition to familiar pastoral interventions into pain, such as being a presence, reading from the Scriptures, and intercessory prayers, some new techniques are being employed, some of them growing out of meditation practices and biofeedback.

One of these is inner visualization, which is described in detail in the books of Carl Simonton, Norman Cousins, and Joseph Dulany.[7] This is a relaxation technique combining deep breathing exercises with autosuggestion, which supports a guided change of perception of the bodily processes which are involved in the pain. By thinking of the area of the body that is painful and developing metaphors and images of what is going on there, it is possible to shift

one's thinking about pain to permit positive interpretations of what is taking place. For example, if the
patient envisions the area of the pain as a sharply
focused spotlight, he or she can visualize the color of
the light changing from a hot, irritated red to a cool,
soothing pale blue. When the painful area is imagined
as the scene of a hostile battle, the image can be shifted
to one of a peaceful area of rest and renewal. The use
of imagery from biblical stories in creative visualization can be helpful for some persons.

This combination of the techniques of meditation
and relaxation, practiced several times daily, has been
shown to be an effective way of reducing pain in many
patients. This approach has the additional advantage
of being something that the patient can do for himself
or herself, after initial guidance and encouragement,
making it a valuable self-help technique for the person
who has felt completely reduced to dependence on
others for care.

Sometimes we say of pain, "I hurt all over," which is
emblematic of the way that pain permeates all
dimensions of our existence. Pain does not involve
just nerve endings; it involves the entire person and
his or her relationship with all that is. This becomes
apparent when people experiencing severe pain try to
interpret it by searching for its meaning. People with a
religious orientation very often try to put their pain
into the context of their relationship with God.
Whether verbalized or not, they may be asking: "Is the
pain a sign of alienation from God?" or, "Is this God's
will for me?" or, "How will God help me to come
through this pain?"

The pastor's task is not to provide ready answers to
such heavy questions. Rather, it is to help the person
explore the questions—what do they mean in terms of
his or her experience? Clichés rarely provide satisfying
answers to such profound existential questions; they
may have superficially described patients' relation-

ships to their centers of meaning in the past, but that was before fierce pain assailed them. Now the search for answers must be done again in the context of pain and approaching death.

In the hospice setting, though a few patients endure continuing severe pain, the majority have their pain controlled by medications administered according to a hospice pattern. While these do not experience the return of pain, they are always aware that their pain-free condition is due to medication and is not their natural bodily state at this time. Although pain may not be a part of their experience at the moment, it is always close enough that the issue of interpreting the possibility of pain is with them. So the pastor continues to be alert for their questions about meaning.

However, the relief which most patients are experiencing is also the basis for hope: not hope for recovery but hope of remaining pain-free. Pastoral care can build upon this hope. Patients have said that this hope of being pain-free also provides them with a resource for facing the end of their lives. They have a sense of being cared for, supported, not only by caregivers but by the very structure of existence. They are not overcome.

The pastoral presence touches the pain that grows out of the patient's sense of being isolated. The feeling that terminal patients have, that no one really understands what they are feeling, can be mitigated by the sensitive pastor who comes from the world of the "healthy" to be with them in their suffering.

A pastor stands with the hospice patient not only as an individual but also as a representative of a faith community. The involvement of the church through aid rendered to the patient by the pastor and fellow parishioners symbolizes the presence of God. The theology the church affirms portrays God as one who is no stranger to pain, but one who suffers along with those who have pain and anguish. The paradigm of Jesus as the Suffering Servant is a powerful image in the Christian community. God's sharing in our suffering is incarnate in the caring community of faith. One's involvement in that community provides not a shield of immunity from pain but a resource for dealing with pain through sharing it.

The way these theological images are interpreted is important. They are not intended to convey that suffering is a normative or ideal way of life or that one is to gain satisfaction through suffering. Rather, they show that suffering is compassionately shared even with the very Source of our being. Persons are never alone in their suffering. This is one of the powerful messages of pastoral care to the hospice patient.

Summary

In spite of the fact that the pain of most hospice patients is effectively controlled medically, this does not mean that the pastoral approach to pain is limited to those situations in which the medicine is not adequate to handle the pain. Knowing, as we do, the part played by anxiety that is related to the possible return of pain and to the stresses that naturally arise in the situation of terminal illness, pastoral caring is an active part of pain control. The effect on the psychological factors of pain is obvious, but it is also possible that pastoral support has a biochemical effect on pain as well.

NOTES

1. Wayne E. Oates and Charles E. Oates, *People in Pain: Guidelines for Pastoral Care* (Philadelphia: Westminster Press, 1985), pp. 14ff.

2. Ibid., pp. 26-27.

3. Ibid., p. 48.

4. Ibid., p. 81.

5. Ibid., p. 117.

6. Ibid., p. 93.

7. Carl Simonton, *Getting Well Again: A Step-by-Step Self-Help Guide to Overcoming Cancer for Patients and Their Families* (Los Angeles: Jeremy P. Tarcher, 1978); Norman Cousins, *The Anatomy of an Illness as Perceived by the Patient: Reflections on Healing and Regeneration* (New York: W. W. Norton, 1979); and Joseph P. Dulany, *We Can Minister with the Dying* (Nashville: Discipleship Resources, 1987).

CHAPTER 5

ISSUES OF BIOMEDICAL ETHICS

Terminality brings one into contact with a number of ethical concerns. In the hospice setting these are also apparent. The pastor who deals with a hospice patient and his or her family may well be queried about the ethical implications of some of the decisions that are being made. Or there may be vague, ill-defined uneasiness about some of the approaches that are involved in hospice care.

It will be helpful for the pastor to have thought through some of these issues in advance. This is not to suggest that the pastor simply "lay down the law" when these concerns arise. Rather, the astute pastoral caregiver will help people try to think through these issues for themselves. Thoughtful preparation on the part of the pastor will enable him or her to discuss freely such issues as trying to control the dying process, abandoning treatment, pain control, possible addiction, and contemplation of suicide. Having considered the complex variables of such issues, the pastor is better equipped to avoid simplistic conclusions or to assert the necessary rightness of his or her own stance.

The pastor's task is further complicated by the fact that not every person in a family is in the same spiritual or ethical position. The patient may be struggling with an issue that is not a major concern for members of the family. Or a family member may disagree with the stance that the patient or another family member is taking. In one hospice situation the wife of the patient suggested withdrawing all medications except for pain relief and "letting him go to heaven," but a son resisted that proposal as "wrong."

In addition to helping each individual to think through the issues, the pastor needs to make a concerted effort to prevent one person from overriding the ethical concerns of another. This means that the pastor will have to be astute in understanding the needs of *all* the persons in the family.

The Ethics of Controlling Life

Some means for controlling life at both its beginning and its ending have been available for centuries. Discussion of the rightness and wrongness of their use is not new either. What appears to have changed, producing the lively debate of our time, is the attitude toward responsible individual participation in the process of living and dying. Employing two terms from the previous chapter on pain, we might say that there has been a shift in many persons' understanding of life from a stoical to a realistic mode.

The ancient Greek Stoics passively submitted themselves to fate. Centuries later, Christian understandings and beliefs, some of which had been infused with Stoic teachings, presented ideal Christian behavior as complete submission to the will of God. Human beings were thus to have a thoroughly passive attitude about both conception and dying. With such a stance, no decision is required other than the decision to be passive.

The realistic mode that predominates today recognizes that means exist for human beings to affect the processes surrounding the beginning and the ending of life. This viewpoint encouraged human beings to be active rather than totally passive, to make decisions based on available opportunities for action. Using simple or elaborate technology, they can decide to affect the processes of living and dying. Medical treatment of any illness is itself such an intervention into the natural processes. This realistic mode of thought is responsible for such common assertions as, "Just as it is all right for a couple to decide whether or not they wish to conceive a child, so it is also acceptable for persons to decide when the quality of life has declined so much that they wish no further life-support technology applied."

Christian understandings can have an impact on this view. Both the available technologies and the human power to make decisions are seen as gifts of divine providence. Human beings are, therefore, properly regarded as endowed by their Creator with intelligence in order to be active participants in life.

Clearly, not everyone in our time holds the same opinion on these crucial issues, and personal views are held with passion. This means that the ethical nature of the questions surrounding the beginning and ending of life are indeed complex, and when hospice patients and families ponder such issues, many turn to their pastors to help them find some useful resolution.

A term often used by families in discussions of such ethical dilemmas is "playing God." Is it right to want to control life or is that playing God, preempting a function rightly belonging to God? One's response to that question depends whether one prefers the stoical or the realistic approach to life.

There is always the possibility of making the wrong decision, but freedom requires that one accept the risk of deciding. The role of the pastor in such situations is that of guide and enabler. It is not to guide persons to a decision that has already been made by the pastor as normative. Rather, it is to guide people through the process of examining the complex medical, personal, ethical, and theological dimensions of their decisions. Thinking through all elements of a decision is infinitely preferable to making decisions impulsively or superficially, or to accepting unthinkingly the decision made by an authority figure.

Another responsibility of the pastor is to assure that decisions are taken voluntarily and not under any compulsion. For the pastor to function effectively, he or she has to have some personal knowledge of both the patient and the family. Personal situations, needs, attitudes, and beliefs have bearing on participation in such decisions. The pastor who does not have some grasp of these variables is operating blindly and with drastically reduced effectiveness.

Many people in our day are trying to anticipate some of the decisions that may be required years hence if they should have a terminal illness. They make a Living Will, deciding that when in the judgment of competent physicians their situation is irreversible and that an acceptable quality of life is no longer possible, they wish no life-prolonging measures to be taken. A growing number of states are now acknowledging that persons have the right to make such decisions. It should be clear that this right must be exercised only voluntarily.

An even more emotional issue in the controlling of the end of life is euthanasia. Here a broad range of options is involved, options which have varying support in the popular mind. They range all the way from not seeking heroic treatment for an illness—to withdrawal of technical life support systems—to withholding medication or nutrition—to cooperating with the patient who wishes to end his or her own life by active means—to ending the life of the person in an effort to spare him or her further suffering.

Some people find all such options unacceptable

because they accept total passivity in such matters as normative. Others will be able to support some or all of the options. Again, it is important for the pastor to help people think through these issues in both the theoretical and the personal ethical dimensions. For example, the husband of a critically ill hospice patient told his pastor: "The other day she was sleeping so soundly after a couple difficult days. The thought crossed my mind: should I just put the pillow over her face and let her rest in peace rather than waking up?" The pastor responded with understanding rather than shock or reproof. He talked with the parishioner about the desperation they were feeling as the illness dragged on and on, about the kind of peace they anticipated, and about the frustration of feeling so powerless and wanting to do something.

Although it is important for our society to discuss rather than to hide from these important issues, hospice is a moderating influence to the debate. In a sense, hospice offers another kind of decision, which is equally valid. By utilizing high level personal caring rather than high-tech medicine, to enable people to live as fully as possible until death occurs, hospice makes some of the choices described above unnecessary. If pain can be controlled, if the dying person can experience the dignity of participating in the decisions affecting treatment and care, if the context of personal relatedness can alleviate isolation and loneliness, more drastic measures to reduce an unacceptable quality of life may not be considered necessary.

The Ethics of Abandoning Treatment

As has already been stated, the very entry of a patient into a hospice program is part of the admission that almost certainly further treatment will not bring a return to health. The patient and the family come to an awareness, which they may or may not be able to articulate, that there is no useful purpose served by continuing treatment. Because this runs counter to a prevailing value in our society that it is wrong to give up, it represents an ethical concern.

The triumphalist ethos that was traced by Frederick Jackson Turner to the frontier spirit that shapes so much of American life is a major cultural value. The westward expansion of American society brought a feeling of being able to conquer any obstacle. There was always another chance to make a fresh start, to find new opportunity, to discover Eldorado. This attitude is deeply engrained in the American spirit.

Behaviorally, it causes Americans to feel that it is somehow wrong to give up, to accept limitation, to abandon the quest for something new and wonderful. Consider the common aphorism, "A winner never quits and a quitter never wins." Only the goals of the quest have changed in time. The Horatio Alger heroes of the capitalism of earlier times may have been supplanted by wizards of technology, but the basic requirements of the quest—persistence, imagination, and money—are the same. Life is lived on the principle that one must not give up.

Our culture also depicts death as an adversary, a concept that is integral to Western, and specifically Christian, thought. Yielding, then, to the enemy can be construed as a kind of treason. Surrender is perfidy. There are those who would see the words of Dylan Thomas, "Rage, rage against the dying of the light," as universally appropriate.[1]

This poses a very real problem for the person who confronts a terminal illness. He or she is faced with the possibility, indeed the necessity, of encountering the ultimate limitation: death. Despite the widespread feeling in recent years that prolonging life in the face of a hopeless situation is absurd (provided that the wishes of the patient are followed), there is still profound uneasiness about giving up hope. Several hospices reported situations in which the patient again and again expressed a wish to die with no further treatment, but family members were insistent that treatment be continued.

Hoping is easier when all is going well. But obstacles to the achievement of goals, hindrances to moving forward, disappointments and defeats, can make hope more difficult. If such limitations are severe, it is possible that periods of hopelessness will result. This is the situation of the hospice patient.

Even in serious illness we struggle with the rightness of giving up hope for a cure. The words "Abandon hope, all ye who enter here," inscribed over the gates of Dante's hell, convey the ultimate in despair. Such hopelessness is linked with the symbolization, deeply rooted in Western culture, of ultimate evil.

Religion and culture are closely intertwined. Within the Christian belief system, hope plays a very important role, so to give up hope may be seen as an indication of lack of trust in the providence of God.

The pastor has a variety of possibilities for helping patients deal with hope. First of all, the nature of hope must be understood. So often it is confused with magical thinking, as if by wishing for something we could bring it into being. Dobihal and Stewart clarify the nature of hope:

> Hope . . . may be seen as different from wishing. To wish for something to be different is a passive emotion and tends to lead toward wanting someone to effect a magical solution. Hope, on the other hand, is a goal-directed vision that enables one to live effectively in the present and move trustingly toward future possibilities.[2]

Hope really accomplishes far more in changing the attitudes and responses of the person who hopes than it does in changing magically the external circumstances of that person's life.

There is a difference between giving up hope and giving up a particular hope. It is a great cruelty to deprive a person of hope. The crucial question is, For what is the person hoping? The task of hospice often involves helping people to work through a transfer of hope from one wish to another, from a hope that is becoming unrealistic to one that has more promise for sustaining the person through the crisis of approaching death.

Sometimes this transfer of hope is from this life to the one to come. In this instance one can give up hope for continued life in the present world and express the hope in new terms of being in a world beyond death.

Others might give up hope in further medical treatment and find it instead in the profound caring of others who will not abandon them to die alone. Hope is transferred from one kind of response to life-threatening illness to another, from medical technology to high-level caring.

Still others might be sustained by the hope that in spite of their death the contributions their lives have made will benefit others. They affirm that life has been worthwhile and that even though their lives end, the process of life goes on. They hope that others will continue to carry on the values that have been contributed or affirmed by their lives.

Pastors who deal with a relatively homogeneous faith community can easily assume that only those who adopt the expression of hope of that church will find comfort in the face of death. However, pastors who are ministering in a more pluralistic setting often make a surprising discovery. They find persons who frame their hope in a way quite different from their faith heritage but are still comforted.

Paul S. Dawson, a hospice chaplain, makes an important observation about this.

I am not convinced that every dying person requires an open-ended future. I have known persons who have faced death calmly with the firm conviction that "it all ends there." But for most, recapitulation emerges as a threshold for a new beginning, transcending the past without losing its essential meaning.[3]

This suggests that a helpful pastoral attitude is to permit the person to express hope in his or her own way rather than to force a particular interpretation on them. While the pastor is free to share the expression of hope that he or she has found most personally meaningful, it must not be presented as normative. The very nature of hope makes such an absolute a contradiction.

The pastor has a function in helping people understand the feelings they have about giving up hope for a cure. While there is great value in understanding also the transfer of hope, an astute pastor will not assume that this transfer is made easily. In the abstract, a person can talk of giving up one hope and finding strength in another. But in actual situations, giving up a hope may be a wrenching experience, even when another form of hope is available.

The inner, personal response to giving up hope is grief. We have long recognized that it is possible to grieve in anticipation of death. We have moved beyond earlier understandings which quantified grief, so that one who grieved 30 percent prior to the death had only 70 percent of grief work to do following the death. Now we recognize that anticipatory grief (although very real) is not the same as grief which takes place following a death, because it does not have the strong sense of finality. There is still some life remaining in the anticipatory situation.

The process of anticipatory grief in the patient begins at the time of diagnosis. This is often followed by a period of treatment which may be effective in slowing the progress of the disease but which in some cases ultimately runs its course and is no longer effective. The patient, the family, and the physician are then faced with the choice of whether or not to continue treatment that is not effective and may be producing difficult side effects. When the decision is made to abandon treatment, the patient enters another dimension of intensity of anticipatory grief, an emotionally moving turning point.

One hospice patient described how she had prayed fervently that the chemotherapy would work, bringing a cure, but then when her physician indicated that there was no improvement and the side effects were becoming increasingly intolerable, she began to pray that the chemotherapy could be ended.

Abandonment of treatment, other than palliative measures, does not mean that everything else is abandoned. Part of the pastoral care function is to help the patient and family to discuss what is being abandoned and what is not. Active therapy is being abandoned. But important human caring-relationships are not being abandoned. The support of hospice personnel is not lost. The pain control measures brought by hospice are not abandoned. Pastoral care is not abandoned.

By the same token, an experience like this can be strengthening rather than totally debilitating if people can see that the willingness to make such crucial decisions is a sign of real strength. One becomes proactive in dealing with the growing crisis of dying not by giving up hope but by realigning one's hopes.

It is so easy to misunderstand poise in the face of death as passivity. The term "relinquishment" has often been used to describe the most helpful attitude for a person confronted with a life-threatening illness. It might be understood as placing oneself in God's hands. It might also be understood as developing a willingness to accept any outcome of the crisis: living on or dying. "Relinquishment" is another way of expressing the ability to make a transition from one hope to another.

Hospice patients and families often have to make "Code" or "No Code" decisions. Medical technology has developed a number of techniques for resuscitating patients who experience cardiac or respiratory arrest. The term "Code" comes from the various code names that are applied to a call for the resuscitation team in the hospital. Their wonderful efforts are to be celebrated when they save the lives of patients who go on to get well. But resuscitation does not seem to be an appropriate response to cardiac or respiratory failure in the hospice patient. Rather than "bringing the person back to life," it tends merely to prolong the inexorable dying process. So hospice families very often have to face a decision: If the patient's heart or breathing stops, do we want to call the resuscitation team (in the hospital) or the ambulance paramedics (in the home) to revive the patient for a few more days of life, or do we simply let him or her go?

It is important that these decisions are reached together by the patient and his or her family, and that the hospice is informed. The pastor may well be asked to assist in unravelling the ethical dimensions of the decision. Although it is somewhat uncommon for families who have gotten to the point of entering a hospice program to have the need to keep the patient alive at all costs, some persons whose own needs make it very difficult for them to give up the patient may not be able to make a "No Code" decision, which is after all a form of relinquishment for the family. They need to be understood and not overpowered by argument to the contrary. The pastor's task is to help them talk about their decision and their understanding about why they are making it. The goal of the pastor is not to compel them to change their minds but to lead them carefully through the decision-making process so that it can be made with as much self-awareness as possible.

Ethical Questions in Pain Control

It seems almost too obvious to point out that the relief of pain is an ethical good. But the issue is not quite so simple. Both our Western heritage and the Christian faith have ennobled suffering. The image of the Suffering Servant is a powerful metaphor in Christian teaching and experience. Scripture is filled with accounts of how persons have been tempered in the fires of suffering. Martyrs have become saints as the result of their suffering.

Some hospice patients and families are so imbued with such belief that they raise ethical questions about pain control. Is it right to free a person totally from pain, when it might be the means for his or her growth? If God has given pain as a means of sanctification, should one interfere with the process?

An even more common stance is based on the assumption that enduring suffering has value in itself. We have great admiration for someone who has endured adversity or pain. Families, following a death, will say with great admiration, "He was so brave . . ."

Having developed the attitude that suffering must somehow have a purpose, some patients and families wonder if interfering with the pain is also interfering with its purpose. Obviously this is not a logical objection, because they will take other steps to modify pain.

The patient's rather than the family's point of view needs to be considered here. The role of the pastor and other hospice caregivers is to help people to talk the question through. If the patient is resolute in accepting the pain, even after talking about it, that wish is honored.

Ethical Questions Related to Taking Narcotics

Some patients and families struggle with the trade-off between relief of pain and taking sizable doses of addicting narcotics. Drug abuse has become a catastrophic problem in our time and rightly receives a great deal of media attention. Public opinion against addiction is growing. A number of pastors interviewed had encountered families, far more frequently than patients, who were concerned that the patient would become an addict as a result of pain control. Again, this is not a very logical argument, because it should be easily recognized that addiction is irrelevant for a person whose life is measured in days or weeks.

Another sort of objection is raised by many formerly self-reliant individuals who see medication, particularly addictive medication, as yet another dependency they would like to resist.

The pastoral caregiver needs to be sensitive to all of these possibilities as he or she relates to patients and families. In those instances where hospice staff encounter resistance to taking prescribed medications, there needs to be exploration and clarification of the underlying reasons for the refusal to follow the pain control plan. The pastor, often perceived as something of an authority on ethical concerns, can help people to talk through their difficulty in recognizing the exceptional nature of hospice care in administering addicting narcotics for effective pain control in the late stages of an illness.

The Ethical Issue of Contemplated Suicide

A patient said to the hospice nurse, "What would happen if I took this whole bottle of pills? Would it put me out of my misery and help me die in peace?" Another patient whose abdomen had filled with fluid asked, "If I lie down, will that make the end come sooner?" Thoughts of suicide are not foreign to many terminally ill patients.

In studies of suicide a broad variety of motivations are described: the need to manipulate the behavior of others by sending a message of desperation, the desire to punish others or oneself, the longing to join a loved one who has already died, the wish to escape from a situation perceived as desperate or intolerable. This last is the most common conscious motivation for those in late-stage terminal illness. It may sometimes be coupled with a wish to spare the family from the ongoing burden of care.

It has been indicated several times that life for the terminally ill person feels out of control. It is not uncommon to find persons in late-stage terminal illness at least wishing for death. Most pastors have encountered parishioners who have said they are praying for death, or who have requested the pastor to offer such a prayer. The ultimate effort at reasserting control over life is the rational contemplation of suicide. The patient chooses to intervene actively in the process of dying. Sometimes the patient is capable of carrying out this intent himself or herself. Other patients may request assistance from family members or friends.

Hospice care may be an effective means for reducing such desires for release. Hospice attempts to re-endow patients with a sense of mastery over their circumstances by encouraging participation in decisions about care. The pain control that can be achieved in most instances and the support which can be given to caring family relationships can do a lot to make the final period of life tolerable at least. But hospice does not work magic. There are a few patients for whom heavy pain remains an issue. There are families who, in spite of massive hospice support, have been so damaged by past relational stresses or emotional impoverishment that they cannot overcome alienation and isolation. Hospice cannot guarantee that no patient will feel sufficiently desperate to contemplate suicide or to carry it out.

There is a broad spectrum of attitudes among pastors toward such suicide. Some would hold that under no circumstances is suicide an acceptable option; it is morally wrong in any setting. (We note that even in the Roman Catholic church, which has consistently maintained a strong position against suicide, in some periods it has been regarded as a permissible choice to avoid rape. Similarly, martyr-dom is affirmed as good, even though a martyr makes the choice to give up life for his or her belief.)

Other pastors would be willing to acknowledge that under certain circumstances and with certain motiva-tions suicide can be a legitimate choice. A criterion which can be applied to such situations is if the decision is based on an affirmation of life as good. Is the patient contemplating suicide in despair, in isolation, in angry protest? Or is the patient, as it were, saying, "This is an act of self-determination in the face of a situation that is increasingly intolerable. I value life but can no longer have an acceptable quality of life. I affirm the value of the life I have lived by drawing to an end the unacceptable quality of the present situation"? Some would confront such a suicide with regret rather than celebration, but would not con-demn it.

Of course, each pastor will reach her or his own stance on the contemplation or carrying out of suicide by a terminally ill parishioner. This stance will affect the way in which the pastor responds to that parishioner. One of the pastors interviewed talked about the situation this way: "I am concerned for what suicide does or can do to the family. I think that if the patient is considering suicide, the family needs to talk about it, so that there is full, mutual understanding of what is being considered. The role of the pastor at this point has to be nurturing, non-directive, non-judgmental." Such an approach sees the issue as one that is approached consciously and rationally rather than impulsively. It recognizes that it involves not only the individual but also those who are part of the family circle. It strongly suggests a resource in family communication and solidarity. It honors the responsible exercise of freedom.

Not every pastor is able to approach that situation from such an open stance. But even the pastor who believes that suicide is not a valid option can respond to the parishioner with understanding and acceptance. To stand over against such a parishioner in shock, disappointment, or judgment for even entertaining the thought of suicide prevents the pastor from offering effective support to the patients in their struggle to improve their quality of life. The pastoral caregiver who can respond empathically to the desperation, the frustration, the pain of the patient contemplating suicide is offering a resource which may make the decision unnecessary.

Ethical Issues in the Care of AIDS Patients

The epidemic of Acquired Immune Deficiency Syndrome has become a concern for hospice programs, because at present all victims of this disease are terminal and many become hospice patients in the late stages of their illness. A few hospices have been set up especially for AIDS patients, but many hospices have cared for AIDS patients. Some ethical considerations have arisen from the patients' care, which the pastor should be prepared to address.

Present medical knowledge indicates that the avenues for transmitting AIDS are limited and that if one is aware of the modes of transmission and avoids them, one can be protected against contagion.

Hospice staffs, like hospital staffs, have been

prepared to deal with AIDS patients through training and sharing of the best available information. By carefully maintaining certain precautionary techniques, the risk of contagion is minimal. However, there is still a *very small* area of calculated risk, which causes concern for some hospice caregivers.

Some hospices make willingness to care for AIDS patients a condition of employment for their staff members; some make such assignments voluntary. This poses some ethical problems to which a pastor may be asked to respond. If one is seriously concerned about contagion, should one risk endangering self and family by caring for an AIDS patient? If one chooses not to accept this responsibility, is one guilty of lack of compassion, as mandated by Christian faith? Such moral dilemmas have been discussed in hospice team conferences. If the pastor is functioning as a member of such a team, she or he may be looked to for guidance.

The function of any leader, pastoral or other, in such a situation is to encourage people to gather the best information available from acknowledged authorities, discuss the questions as rationally as possible, and preserve the right of caregivers to make informed voluntary commitments.

Another dimension of ethical concern in caring for AIDS patients is raised by the fact that many in our country contracted the disease through homosexual contacts. Some persons with strong feeling toward the gay community have interpreted AIDS as a sign of divine retribution. Others regard the epidemic as a way of discouraging homosexual relationships through fear of contagion. Still others are able to respond to these patients' needs, quite apart from their opinions about the homosexual life-style.

A hospice worker interviewed on the West Coast observed, "Many of our AIDS patients have very much wanted to go back to their church of origin, even though they may have left it because they felt excluded in the past." Many gay persons feel they are no longer acceptable in their home churches. They may affiliate with gay churches, but the crisis of dying of AIDS creates in them a desire to renew contact with their old church home. There can be a number of possible motives for such a desire. The person may be seeking reconciliation, the restoration of an accepting relationship. The person may be responding to the need for the familiar and the stable in a situation filled with profound disequilibrium.

The pastoral caregiver facing such a situation will find that it is not enough to simply "welcome a penitent sinner back home." Rather, the pastor should make a gracious response, directed primarily to a terminally ill person in need of care and support, and only secondarily to a person who happens to be gay. Grace in the Christian tradition has always meant *unconditional* love. This is the highest ethical stance.

Issues of Truth-Telling and Informed Consent

Authority structures have been questioned everywhere in our contemporary society, and medical authority has not been immune to this. The former pattern is passé: not bothering to inform a patient of his or her situation, of the treatments prescribed, and of the real or potential risks involved, because the physician is going to make all the decisions. Many instances can be cited from the past in which truth-telling was considered harmful and produced a bad experience for the patient, but this assumed a totally passive patient.

Hospice and its openness in dealing with approaching death has been one component in a new concern for truth-telling. It is important to recognize hospice's commitment to *two* things: that the truth be told openly and that it be told in a context of caring and support that does not leave the persons desolate. It is well demonstrated in the work of Kübler-Ross, Saunders, and others that most patients already strongly suspect the truth; their greatest need is for someone who will listen as they talk about their concerns, their fears, their hopes, their resources.[4]

In the past there have been discussions about whether or not the pastor should be involved in telling persons their situation. Generally it has been assumed that this is the primary responsibility of the attending physician. Pastors, however, have found themselves in very awkward positions when patients have not been told the truth about their conditions.

Hospice supports openness in dealing with the terminal nature of an illness, in letting the patient indicate her or his wishes to know rather than having an authority figure decide what is or is not good for the patient, and in seeing truth-telling as a function of a team that operates collegially rather than hierarchically. Such limitations on pretense and deception have made the pastor's relationship to the patient and family much more productive.

The basis for decisions about truth-telling rests in part on accurate assessment of the patient's resources for dealing with the situation. The pastor often has an advantage of prior acquaintance with the patient and is in a position to make a major contribution to the hospice team's assessment of the patient's resources. The pastor's ethical commitment to the right of the patient to be in touch with the reality of his or her situation, a commitment often shared by others, suggests that the pastor can advocate for the patient's right to know. This is accompanied by the pastor's commitment to enabling the patient to have and use all available resources. Hospice so clearly shows that truth-telling should always operate in the context of caring relationships manifest in physical, emotional, and spiritual support.

101

One hospice patient described his situation as moving from "red hope" to "pale pink hope," when the physician indicated that chemotherapy had proved unsuccessful and serious new metastases had been found. The pastor focused on that metaphor in the first of several family conversations about how they might deal with the weeks ahead. Although they no longer could hope for a cure, they could hope for some good days together, with pain control, the support of the hospice staff and friends, and deepening faith.

There is another side to this ethical commitment to truth-telling. There must be a similar commitment to permitting the patient to adopt a stance which is not normative for hospice patients. Hospice and the pastoral caregiver do not have the right to manipulate persons into dying good deaths. It is a truism that each person dies his or her own death.

A good bit of the literature on dying that has developed in recent years produced this normative expectation for "good" dying. The "right" way to die is to be fully accepting of one's approaching death, to be supported by a family which is motivated by perfect love for one another, to live each remaining day triumphally, and to be assisted by a hospice staff operating with total efficiency in meeting every need. Such an ideal has sometimes been taken as a mandate to try to press people into that mold, whether they fit or not.

The pastor can be a particularly helpful resource at this point because this is an issue with which she or he is quite familiar. The Christian faith community has an ideal for living. At the same time it recognizes that the ideal is not achievable. Christian theology strongly emphasizes that salvation comes by grace, not by obsessive pursuit of the ideal; persons are accepted as they are, not as they are supposed to be. The familiarity of the pastor with this theological model should enable a helpful understanding in hospice that patients are to be accepted as they are and helped to die their own deaths, rather than pushing them to achieve the normative ideal.

Pastoral caregivers have to recognize that they too can easily fall into this trap. Some of the older, more mechanical understandings of what it meant to be "prepared to die" ran this risk. People were expected to think the right thoughts and say the right words in order to be ready to die. Pastors were sometimes disappointed or judgmental when parishioners did not or could not meet these expectations, when pillars of the church confronted death with real anxiety or with bitter anger. A commitment to the experience of grace, on the other hand, starts with people as they are and accepts them in their individuality.

Ethical Issues in the Hospice "Contract"

One of the pastors interviewed pointed to an ethical concern that is easily missed in providing hospice care. He questioned the right of hospice to intervene in families beyond the contract to deal with the terminal illness.

Because of the comprehensive and holistic understanding of patients and families, it is easy to establish legitimate connections between the process of dying and the whole gamut of family relationships. The access that hospice has to intimate family settings by, for instance, entering homes and participating in family relationships, offers the possibility of becoming involved in family issues only tangentially related to the dying of the patient. Does hospice have the right to deal on its own initiative with the alcoholism of a family member, or delinquent behavior, or mismanagement of family finances?

It is possible to understand hospice care as making a contract with a patient and her or his family to help them to cope with the approaching death. This is the explicit understanding of the family. The pastor in the interview argued that, even with the best of intentions, hospice sometimes violated the contract by becoming involved in domestic problems and other concerns when no permission had been given by the family for hospice to deal with such issues. He argued that admission to hospice was not a license to become involved in every aspect of the experience of the patient and family. Such interventions could be made ethically only upon invitation of the family or patient. The pastor has the right to raise questions if such an extension of hospice concerns occurs.

Summary

Hospice care is founded on values of individuality, of autonomy, and of dignity. It provides services but it is also concerned with questions about the motivations that lie behind the caregiving. For these reasons ethical issues in hospice care have to be considered. Without suggesting that ethics is the exclusive province of the clergy, it is true that training and experience make the pastor, as a participant in hospice care, a resource for dealing with the profound issues involved in helping patients and families deal with terminal illness.

NOTES

1. Dylan Thomas, "Do not go gentle into that good night," *Collected Poems* (New York: New Directions, 1957), p. 128.

2. Edward F. Dobihal, Jr., and Charles William Stewart, *When a Friend is Dying* (Nashville: Abingdon Press, 1984), p. 84.

3. Paul S. Dawson, "Reflections of a Hospice Chaplain," in *A Hospice Handbook*, eds. Michael Hamilton and Helen Reid (Grand Rapids: Eerdmans, 1980), p. 71.

4. Elisabeth Kübler-Ross, *On Death and Dying* (New York: Macmillan, 1969), chapter 2; Cicely Saunders, "Telling Patients," *District Nursing* (Sept. 1965): 149-54.

CHAPTER 6

HOME CARE AND THE FAMILY AS THE UNIT OF CARE

Hospice will provide care for the terminally ill person and his or her family wherever those persons are or wish to be or can afford to be. Almost all hospice programs are prepared to care for patients and families in both the home setting and in an in-patient facility.

Since self-determination is one major significant principle in hospice care, the decision about where care will be given is made primarily by the patient and family. It is the role of hospice to help people to appraise realistically their situation, as well as understanding the emotional dynamics that go into the decision making.

A number of factors, both negative and positive, contribute to this decision. The quality of family relationships is of primary importance. Neither terminal illness nor hospice care will repair deep fractures in family structure. A family with significant relational problems will have difficulty with home care and will probably be better served in an in-patient setting, where full-time staff can serve a surrogate family role in the care of the patient. Where there are negative or neutral family relationships, there may be a preference for distancing from the patient in preparation for the death. Other families may prefer to share the experience of helping the patient live out the remainder of his or her days in the intimacy of the family circle at home. Those families respond positively to the patient's wish to die at home and with the support of hospice services are able to provide the care that makes it possible.

For some families, economic factors are an important consideration in the decision, especially if family finances have been depleted by long illness and treatment, or if insurance benefits are not available for hospice care. Obviously, home care is the most economical. In-patient hospice care is less expensive than regular hospital care because certain ancillary hospital services are not required. Hospice has a responsibility to help people understand the economic realities of their situations and to put them in touch with available resources, both private and public. Most hospices will provide care without regard for the family's ability to pay.

It has been found in the National Hospice Study reported by the Hastings Center that the kind of service most readily available through a given hospice program has a bearing on the decision.[1] Hospices that have an integral relationship with an in-patient facility care for the majority of their patients on an in-patient basis. Those programs that only contract with hospitals or convalescent facilities care for the majority of patients in their homes. Intentionally or unintentionally, then, the institutional pattern of the hospice available in the community is a factor in the decision about where care is given. Only a few very large cities have more than one hospice available, so there are not a variety of patterns available for the majority of hospice patients.

There may not be consensus in the family about where care can best be given, which is important since the effectiveness of hospice care depends on agreement between the patient and those family members upon whom most of the responsibility will rest as to whether care should be at home or in-patient. The pastor may play a role in the development of the necessary consensus by helping people understand all the options open to them and facilitating real openness in talking about wishes and hesitancies.

The pastor often may be in a better position than hospice staff, because of longer acquaintance with the family, to work with the dynamics of interpersonal relationships that are either complicating or enabling the decision process. There are sometimes strong feelings on the part of the patient or significant members of the family, which need to be dealt with as decisions are made about whether to seek hospice care and in what setting it should be delivered. One pastor was helpful to hospice by describing a long-standing power struggle between adult children of the hospice patient, which was complicating the decision-making process because whatever one suggested the other opposed. Together the pastor and the hospice staff worked to empower the patient to make decisions for herself instead of being a victim of the inability of her children to reach a consensus.

Patients Who Feel Burdensome to Their Families

A number of the pastors interviewed report that they have encountered these feelings in parishioners. "I hear patients apologizing to their families for putting them through this." "Patients say, 'I just don't want to feel like a burden.' "

Good communication is an essential ingredient in trying to deal with such situations. The patient needs to be free to express himself or herself honestly and openly. It is a normal social tendency to try to cover up such feelings or to minimize them. Patients will be told, "Now, don't you talk that way. Of course, you are not a burden." That does not solve the problems but only assures that it cannot be talked about.

The pastor will begin by empathically responding to the patient, indicating that it is quite understandable not to want to be dependent, a burden on others. One pastor put it this way: "I admit to them right away that they are a burden but affirm that this is a matter of circumstance not intention. It's phoney to say, 'You're not a burden,' when the heavy load on the family is so obvious. I'd much rather help people talk about it openly than encourage them to sweep it under the rug." Another pastor said, "People do feel like a burden initially, but when they see the support coming through hospice, they see that it can be done."

Once the patient is assured that her or his concern is perfectly understandable, that it is an expression of loving concern for the family, and that it is okay to have such feelings, some other points of view can be offered. Family members may be able to express sincerely their willingness to provide care. They may be able to interpret their care as a gift to the patient, rather than an obligation.

Sometimes communication is aided by asking the patient to think in terms of reversed roles: How would he or she respond if the situation were turned around? One needs some background knowledge of the patient and the family dynamics before using such an approach. It might assist a family that has considerable resources for caring, but it could be counterproductive in a situation where the patient is not at all sure if he or she could assume the role of caregiver if the situation were reversed.

This suggests that an important variable is the extent to which the patient's worries convey a sense of personal worthlessness. Does the patient feel like a burden because he or she has a low self-image of long standing, or is depressed? To argue with such a view of self or to try to talk a person out of feeling depressed very often only deepens the sense of isolation. An approach of more substantive counseling, pastoral or other, would be a necessary prelude to changes in the person's feeling of being a burden.

In the absence of such a sense of worthlessness, hospice care very often relieves the initial fear of being a burden. Once the support system is explained and is in place, people find that they can function quite effectively. Hospice works. If there is a willingness on the part of some family members and if there is enough physical and emotional stamina, the situation turns from feelings of helplessness to helpfulness.

Families Who Can't Handle Home Care

Clearly, there are some families that do not have the physical or emotional resources to give extensive home care. An aged spouse of the patient may really want to provide care but may not have the stamina to do it. Or family members may be so anxious about the approaching death that they are immobilized. Coping mechanisms that have functioned in the past are felt to be inadequate for the present crisis.

When pastors were asked how they deal with such situations, three representative responses were "My primary concern is that the patient not feel rejected," "I wouldn't tell families what to do," and, "I would not lay guilt on them." All of these pastoral concerns are valid. They show that the pastor has more responsibility to the persons involved than to shaping the situation.

This suggests that careful attention has to be given to the psychological makeup of the persons involved before beginning a problem-solving approach. If family reluctance to provide home care is simply due to lack of information about all the kinds of support hospice can provide, giving that information removes the obstacle. But if there are deep psychological reasons for their reluctance, such as anger, anxiety, hostility, or guilt, those obstacles need to be talked about before putting full reliance on the support hospice can give. It may be that deep-seated feelings like these cannot be dealt with completely before deciding where hospice care will be given, but preliminary discussion can begin a counseling process that can go on while hospice care is being given in either the home or an in-patient facility.

Hospice staff members and pastors, who have seen hospice support operate, know how participation in that support can be a real asset not only in caring for the patient but also in dealing with the feelings and self-images of the family members. This knowledge, however, cannot be allowed to short-circuit the process through which family members work through the obstacles to being willing to provide home care.

It is important for them and for hospice to know why they are having problems with home care. Many families haven't been exposed to death before and the thought of being close to a dying person or being present when death occurs is frightening to them. Support relieves much anxiety that is purely situational. A deeper counseling process may be needed to work with the fear of their own deaths—that anxiety which Tillich described as "the threat of non-being."

Hospice is concerned for both the patient and the family. If there are deep reasons for the inability of family members to provide care to the patient, no one will be well-served by trying to compel them to do what they cannot. People have to be supported in looking to their own well-being, not in the interest of self-centeredness but of effective, comprehensive care.

Experience has shown that many people find psychological benefit, both before and after the death of the patient, from being involved with care. If the hesitancies of family members are situational rather than intrapersonal, it can be shown that hospice can mobilize many resources to help them provide home care. Families are given permission to do what they think best. Even when home care is not a suitable option, the role of the pastor and hospice staff is to develop the process of family communication so that the patient will feel a great deal of family involvement, even in the in-patient setting.

A home-care hospice has to know when it is time to remain at home no longer. Family resources which functioned well at the begnning of hospice care may be depleted. Physical and emotional fatigue can develop. Sometimes the pastor is in a good position to sense whether families are beginning to approach their limits. By discussing this with hospice staff, a response to their needs can be made. A short hospitalization can be arranged to provide respite for the family, or home care may be terminated and hospice care shifted to an in-patient facility.

Pastors have a particular role in dealing with the guilt that may arise from home-care issues. Family members who simply do not feel comfortable with home care may feel very guilty because they are not able to perform satisfactorily the proper role of spouse, son, or daughter. When a patient has to be transferred to a hospital, even with very good reason, many families are apologetic and feel guilt. They wanted to continue to provide home care, but could not.

A sense of being judged, either by self or others, is not uncommon in such situations. This stood out in the bereavement support group of one hospice, in which a real conflict developed between those mourners who had cared for their patient at home and those who, for a variety of reasons, had not chosen to do so. The bereavement counselor had to work with the perceptions of persons in both groups: the assumed, and somewhat judgmental, sense of superiority of those who provided home care and the defensive guilt of those who did not. A pastor will have to be alert to such dynamics and be helpful in enabling people to talk about them.

A particular form of guilt is frequently seen when a patient lingers on and on, far exceeding the prognosis. A responsibility that was accepted in the belief that it would last only a few weeks or months, now extends to many months. Tremendous ambivalence results. On one hand family members are glad that the patient still lives, especially if some quality of life remains. But at the same time, they have begun to adjust to thoughts of life without the presence of the patient and are ready to begin reconstructing their lives under that new situation. They begin to experience anger and guilt as a result of these mixed feelings.

Pastors, more than any of the other professionals dealing with hospice patients and families, have time-honored ways of helping people deal with guilt: catharsis, confession, expression of regret, repentance, understanding and acceptance in spite of real or imagined deficiency, forgiveness. A pastor is well reminded of a truism from Calvin's *Institutes*: Grace precedes repentance. A person can only confront his or her guilt in a context of grace, knowing that forgiveness is possible. This is quite different from the frequent assumption that repentance comes only after conviction through accusation or judgment. Calvin reminds us that love is judgment, and that acceptance and understanding are the most fruitful context for helping people deal with their guilt. This is one of the situations where it is highly desirable for the pastor to be working closely with the hospice staff in dealing with issues of home care.

The Benefits of Home Care

If one of the goals of hospice care is to enable people to live as fully as possible the weeks and days that remain to them, this happens most easily in places that can be regarded as the normal setting for life, or, more accurately, the setting for "normal living." Normalcy is relative, of course, but hospice does everything it can to keep elements of the normal in the lives of patients and families.

Home is the most familiar context of our living. Unless there are exceptionally negative circumstances, "Home is where the heart is." At home people are more comfortable, more relaxed, more apt to be surrounded by caring family members.

Being cared for at home helps many patients to deal with the common fear that they will be alone when they die. It is not a guarantee, because death can come unexpectedly, when no one is at the patient's bedside. But hospice experience would show that because family members are around most of the time, it is more likely that they will be with the patient at the time of death.

Corollary to this is the patients' wish to be in familiar surroundings which contain many mementoes of their lives. Patients do not feel comfortable in the strange setting of an in-patient facility, no matter how nice it might be. They are inserted temporarily into that setting, whereas at home they "belong."

In a hospital or nursing home, there are many institutional regulations and procedures that must be followed. Patients are passive ingredients in the system. Even close family members are "VISITORS." They go to unfamiliar places to visit the patient. They park in a visitors' area. They abide by visitors' rules, even though these may be relaxed for dying patients. All of these very natural and understandable distinctions are reminders that normal family relationships are not operative in this setting.

Home is a place where we are accustomed to being actively involved in the processes of living. Patients and their families are more clearly in control. They can come and go from the patient without parking difficulties, without having to be quiet out of consideration for other patients, without constant reminders of the hierarchical authority system of the health care facility.

Closure is accomplished more effectively in a setting full of the familiar than in an in-patient setting where people already feel detached. Of course, closure is not impossible in a hospital setting, but it is often much easier and more natural in the home where one is literally surrounded by the people and things one loves.

Pastoral Care and the Home Setting

Because pastors want to deal with real persons rather than *personae*, the pastoral relationship is stronger in a setting where the identity of the parishioner is reinforced by the pressure of the artifacts of his or her life: personal belongings, pictures, favorite chairs, hobbies—the symbolic representations of the person. These are not simply "conversation starters," but extensions of the personhood of the parishioner. At a time when people may be more introspective than usual, there is value in having the visual supports that help show what this person is really all about.

Many pastors interviewed affirmed that it is easier for them and for patients to talk about death in the natural setting of the home. Both can be more relaxed in familiar surroundings; the home setting insures privacy, which facilitates deeper self-disclosing conversation. They also felt that they had more access to family members, because in the hospital the family might not be there when the pastor calls.

Several pastors who were interviewed suggested that they felt more comfortable and effective in the home setting because in hospitals they felt like adjuncts to the whole system. Some pastors said that the routine of the hospital frequently interrupted meaningful dialogue. Because hospital staff had the obligation to care for many patients, they understandably found it difficult not to interrupt pastoral conversations to provide routine or prescribed care.

A few pastors indicated that, while they saw the value of home care, they found it added to their workload. Like physicians, they saw "house calls" as less convenient and more time consuming. One pastor commented that the extensive involvement of family members, volunteers, and others in the care of the patient at home interfered with pastoral care, but this was not a problem for most pastors.

The home setting also facilitates a pastor's working with the anticipatory grief of both patient and family. It permits a more gradual, inclusive process of mourning. A pastor suggested, "The fact that care is given at home surrounds the patient and family with an environment full of little 'emotional triggers' that permit grief to be dealt with in manageable increments."

Hospice and Concern with the Family
(Home or In-patient Setting)

In the hospice approach families not only are caregivers, they also receive a great deal of care. Death affects not only the terminally ill patient but also the family because they are undergoing an experience of loss, both before and after the clinical death of the patient. So hospice focuses considerable attention on members of the family as well as on the patient.

Many hospices, particularly those which emphasize home care, require as a condition for admission the involvement of a primary careperson. Most often this is a member of the family but it can be a surrogate family member—a friend. Although such a hands-on caregiver is not essential when the hospice patient is in a hospital or nursing home setting, the involvement of family is important nevertheless, both as givers and receivers of care. The emotional support, the sense of belonging, the opportunity to talk seriously in face of the separation that is imminent, are important both for the dying patient and the family.

This concern for the family begins at the point of admission to a hospice program. The family is immediately involved in decision making: Will treatment in hope of cure be abandoned? Will care be given at home or in the hospital? How will responsibilities be shared? It becomes clear very quickly that the family is shifting from a passive, partially informed status to participatory involvement. This is not dumped on them but is done in a context of very practical support. Hospice is there to help them take on this new role.

The pastoral caregiver needs to be alert to ways of helping parishioners make this transition. To accept and participate in change always requires faith. The pastor does not minimize the anxiety that can accompany the possibility of change, but points to a resource that enables people to venture into the fearful unknown.

The onset of responsibility for care can be very disconcerting for the family. Some people are accustomed to providing the kind of care required, but for many others it is a new and anxiety-producing experience. Hospice staff are prepared to train people for unfamiliar tasks. Where people are unable or unwilling to take on the responsibilities of physical care, hospice provides as much of that care as possible.

Hinton writes, "If, together with adequate physical care, the dying person had sufficient human companionship, most of his anguish would be prevented. He wants to see and know that those about him still have a warm interest in himself."[2] This is one of the surest ways to provide quality of life. The holistic focus of hospice on patient needs makes family support a crucial ingredient of hospice care. The acceptance of approaching death is made easier because it is a shared experience in the family.

So, in addition to training in nursing care, professional and non-professional hospice caregivers model many attitudes and behaviors which family members can adopt in response to the situation in which they find themselves: openness, honesty, respect for individuality, communication, calmness. No one is compelled to follow this modeling, but it is there as an indicator of how help can be both given and received.

Those who are totally unfamiliar with hospice care might think this honest confrontation of approaching death a terribly morbid and pessimistic preoccupation, as if the family were talking about death twenty-four hours a day. Experience shows that most often, once openness about the death is established people are freed for much more relaxed, natural conversations about everyday living.

Hospice tries to help people begin to let go of their loved one. As we have already indicated, the grieving process for the family is already going on while they are caring for the patient. This is a complex situation because, on one hand, as Liston Mills points out, "A . . . common problem for families is the feeling of abandonment and the ways this complicates their grief work and their relation to the patient. Not only is the patient leaving them but if the illness is of any duration friends also begin to neglect them so that they are left alone to deal with their grief."[3] On the other hand, they need to begin, emotionally, to let go.

Hospice tries to help people deal with these contradictory feelings, feeling abandoned and simultaneously needing to let go, by providing supportive care to the family prior to the patient's death and explaining its intention to continue providing care for the family after the death. One hospice family wrote in a letter of appreciation for hospice care: "One of the things that kept us going was our awareness that hospice would never give up its concern for us as a family."

Just as the patient is helped by being surrounded by family, there is support in ongoing contact with friends. Hospice wants to encourage their participation. If the setting is home care, friends can be in and out of the home as they were before the onset of the illness. The candor with which approaching death is acknowledged through hospice helps ease these relationships. One patient said, "Because friends know that I'm going to die, it is easier to relate."

Pastoral Care and the Patient and Family

Unlike many other professions that focus sharply on the person with the problem and tangentially on the family of that person, pastors have always provided care in the family context, where it exists. As already pointed out, this is similar to the style and form of hospice care, except that the pastor has probably known the family prior to the onset of the crisis of terminal illness. Joining the pastor to the hospice team often provides a longitudinal view of the family which can be an advantage to all the caregivers. If there is a concern for confidentiality of pastoral relationships, persons can be asked for permission to share professionally certain insights about past family dynamics, in the interest of better hospice care.

Because of the close relationship of church and family in the traditions of our society, it is easy for families to see that the pastor is a direct caregiver for all of them, not just for the patient. Without implying a negative judgment, reflect on how different this is from medical practice. When a physician is seeing a patient, it is very clear that the person is the only one being treated; the physician's professional responsibility extends to family members only to the extent that they have an effect on the patient's condition. This is not to imply that physicians are uncaring, but that their professional responsibilities are clearly defined in that way by our society.

The pastor in the hospice setting should be committed to spending some quality time with patients and their families. Hasty, perfunctory visits are not in order. National standards for hospice care indicate that a full-time hospice nurse should have a caseload of seven patients. Simple arithmetic would indicate that each patient should receive an average of five hours of the nurse's time each week. Just as nurses who work in hospice programs are able to spend much more time on a visit with a patient than they would as Visiting Nurses or as nurses in the hospital, the pastor should budget larger amounts of time to be available to hospice patients and families. Of course, this is subject to the wishes of the patient and family, but at least the pastor can make clear that the time is available.

Unhurried visits enable the pastor both to be alert for particular spiritual needs in the patient and family and to foster a more intense response. There is less temptation to offer a perfunctory prayer or to quote a familiar scripture in lieu of thoughtful conversation that encourages persons to express the depths of their concerns.

Of course, this is not a warrant to impose pastoral visits on anyone. The patient or family members may not want as much time as the pastor is willing to give, or they may not find the visit as helpful as the pastor thinks it is. The pastor needs to be extremely alert to nonverbal signals that the person does not wish the visit to go on. It may be a good idea to discuss the matter of visits with the parishioner. Hopefully, the openness encouraged by hospice and the degree to which people are supported in deciding for themselves what care they most need will also make possible an honest negotiation of pastoral visits.

It is vital that visits be relevant to patient and family needs. One of the pastoral caregivers interviewed uses a very effective approach. She said that she verbalizes to patients and families what she is feeling during her visit. She might say, "I am feeling a great deal of love here today," or, "I am feeling a lot of stress in what is happening today." This approach frees both the pastor and the parishioners to talk at a feeling level. It provides a unique access to spiritual concerns that may be hard to verbalize.

Pastoral visits also contribute to hospice support of the patient by providing an avenue for communication of special needs, which the pastor can share with the hospice team. Often the pastor, through the church, can help meet needs for respite care, for some help with household duties, and for companionship for a member of the family who is feeling stress.

The stress brought on by serious illness and its consequences involves many factors: worry and anxiety, fatigue produced by long hours of physical caregiving, inability to get away for some periods of relaxation. It is further complicated by the disruption of the family through necessary redistribution of responsibilities and a shifting of authority roles within the family structure. This can destabilize the family at a time when its resources are most needed.

The pastoral caregiver will be alert to these changes and will give people the opportunity to talk about them. One spouse may have to take over completely the role which the patient-spouse had always fulfilled. Home care may bring about a role reversal, in which an adult child may have to take over parental functions, even to dealing with a patient's personal care: bathing, dressing, assisting to the toilet or bedpan. These can be occasions of great tenderness, but they also can be highly disconcerting for both the patient and the caregiver. They produce discomfort, embarrassment, reminders of the shifting equation of strength and weakness. These are emotional experiences. The pastor will be available to help people talk about their reactions to such changes in their family lives: their discomforts, their anger and frustration, their anxiety, their joy. To reach the point where such concerns can be sensitively discussed requires that the pastor will have spent enough time to develop a personal as well as a professional relationship.

Another dimension of pastoral caregiving recognizes that it is virtually impossible to be caught up in a highly charged life situation like terminal illness without feeling some guilt. The human condition of imperfection means that we err again and again in our interpersonal relationships. When terminality underlines the brevity of life and produces a kind of "bottom line" motif, it is virtually impossible not to feel regret and guilt over the flaws in even the strongest relationships. As Wentzel reminds us:

> The problem of guilt is expressed in every decision families have to make for the well-being of a patient. Never knowing what is absolutely the best thing to do, partly because their own best interests are involved, they are always confronted with the question of what might have been if other choices had been made. Anxiety over guilt is also a major block in the bereavement process for survivors who try to do for the deceased what they did not or could not do for him while he was still alive.[4]

The pastor is no stranger to such perceptions. His or her understanding will provide a lot of space for thoughtful, caring people to express their guilt.

The pastoral caregiver needs to be particularly sensitive to the guilt felt by family members who are not able to provide home care or by those who botch the job even with all the support hospice can give. Often this is perceived as the ultimate breakdown of familial relationships, even in loving families.

Pastoral care does not try to dilute guilt by explaining it away. It is real to the person and must be confronted as such. The role of the pastor is neither to induce nor to reduce guilt. It is to deal with guilt in the ways in which the Christian faith community has always dealt with it. It is helped to expression, is talked about, is translated from looking at a particular human behavior to seeing that behavior in the light of the human situation. The remedy is presented not as trying harder to undo actions but as accepting love and understanding. The pastor is an active communicator of this process.

Continuing Parish Activity as Pastoral Caring

The pastor is often the only person of the hospice team who brings along a functioning community to which the patient and family relate. Frequently the patient in the early stages of hospice care is still able to be up and about. Attendance at worship and meetings of church groups is quite possible. Unfortunately, many in our society still wish to deny death and, therefore, prefer to keep the dying out of sight.

Patients who are still mobile and their families should be encouraged to continue participating in the life of the congregation, attending worship as long as they are able. Not only does this provide a way for relating as part of a group to the primary resource of spiritual strength, but it also puts the patient physically in the midst of a caring, responding community. There is no good reason why the church, which publicly celebrates so many of the great moments of life, limits its participation in the final phase of life to a funeral. The pastor can provide a great deal of encouragement for dying persons and their families to remain involved in the life of the church as long as possible. Once the patient is no longer able to attend, this encouragement should still be extended to families and appropriate respite care arranged so that they can attend services or other meetings. Such activity reduces their sense of isolation and keeps them related to a community which will offer a resource during the period of readjustment following the death.

Dobihal and Stewart point out that certain special features of the worship life of the congregation should be made available to hospice patients and their families.

> Many significant acts of life are carried out within the corporate Body [the Church], and it is important to see whether any of those events need to be lived out by the dying person before death. Is there to be a marriage, a baptism, a confirmation? Is the person waiting for Christmas, Easter? The calendar may need to be changed, usually moved up a bit. The service may have to be adapted slightly.[5]

The willingness of the church, through the pastor, to be flexible in such ways is effective testimony to the importance of such high moments in the life of the community and to the caring nature of the community.

Prayers, eucharist or communion, and anointing are channels of pastoral care, providing not only spiritual but also psychological and social support. They offer an excellent opportunity to draw a family together. We have been so imbued with the view of our society that religion is a private matter that we often miss opportunities to express the corporate nature of worship and sacrament. The pastoral caregiver should see the liturgical desirability and the psychological value to making acts of pastoral care family rituals. The hospice emphasis on the family as the unit of care provides an important reminder to the pastoral caregiver to see pastoral care in the family context, rather than as a private ministry to the dying person.

Dealing with Difficult Patients or Families

Hospice is a very human venture; staff members, patients, and families have their imperfections. Hospice is no different from the normal arena of the pastor's activity.

Our focus here is on just one of the dimensions of those imperfections. There do occur in hospice instances when it is very onerous for staff members and the pastor to deal with particularly difficult situations or people. Caregivers find that they have to drive themselves to become involved in certain settings because of the problems they encounter there.

Sometimes it is a purely circumstantial matter: extremely unpleasant physical circumstances. It may be an extremely dirty, smelly house. It may be very unpleasant sights or smells that result from the patient's condition. It may be an urban neighborhood in which one feels very alien, even threatened.

Other times it is the people who pose the difficulty. Either as a result of long-term personal style or under the stress of the terminal illness, patients or family members can become very demanding and unreasonable. Or they may be highly manipulative persons who alienate the caregiver. There may be so much anger and hostility that it is displaced on any convenient target, even the potential helper. Or it may be that people are so limited in intelligence or so poorly organized that they repeatedly fail to follow instructions for providing the care that is needed. Such difficulties produce great frustration in hospice caregivers, reducing their effectiveness and often causing them to reproach themselves for their failure to cope with the difficulty.

The pastoral caregiver has a number of possible responsibilities in such situations. There continues to be a responsibility to the dying patient and family. Pastoral care will involve trying to understand what is going on, why people are reacting as they are. One tries to respond to the underlying needs by offering caring and acceptance.

The son of a patient was having great difficulty letting go of his mother. She wanted so much for the end to come, even to the point of refusing to eat. Her son was unwilling to abandon treatment, insisting on taking the patient to a large medical center for heroic experimental treatment. He wanted to do everything to keep her alive. She wanted to die. There was very little effective communication between them. The pastoral caregiver intervened by exploring very intentionally with the son the difficulty he was having allowing his mother to die. He was able to share some strong negative feelings he had harbored for some years toward his mother. With the support and direct involvement of the pastor, he was able to talk with his mother about the events which had produced those feelings. They worked out a sufficient resolution to permit the son to admit that it would be a good thing for his mother to be at rest rather than to continue the struggle to survive.

At times pastoral care must be confrontative, pointing out in love, not anger, what appears to be going on and asking people to consider the consequences of their behavior, or refusing to be manipulated. It must be clear that this is being done in an effort to help the persons deal with their situation, rather than out of rejection.

The pastoral caregiver may also have a responsibility to other helpers, if access is possible. As one of the pastors interviewed said, "Failure to make a difference is very stressful for caregivers." It is not unusual for helpers to feel guilty in such situations: "I should be able to handle this."The pastor will also have to deal with her or his own responses to apparently unsuccessful interventions. Self-image, both personal and professional, can be badly bruised in settings where patient and family resistance produces in the pastor anger rather than compassion, or where every obvious attempt to help is frustrated. Dealing with families in highly stressful circumstances can easily pose such problems.

The interdisciplinary team is a most helpful resource in these situations. Team members can discuss their reactions and call on the competencies of a variety of disciplines to find support for trying to continue to relate and to change difficult situations. For example, in the case of the son who could not allow his mother to die, a number of members of the team were involved. A staff nurse raised the problem in a weekly team conference. The medical director discussed the patient's prognosis and the miniscule chances for its improvement, even with the heroic treatment. The pastor was able to talk about both the patient's wish to die and the son's difficulty in letting go. Not only did the team mutually work through the situation, they also shared their frustration and anger.

Children in the Home

The family as the unit of care and, when acceptable, the home as the place of care make the approach of hospice inclusive rather than exclusive. Family members are involved rather than being passive or isolated. This does not refer only to adult members of the family.

Studies done on death and bereavement in recent years emphasized that some unhealthy and unhelpful approaches have developed in dealing with children when there is a death in the family. The fragmentation of the family, the lack of experience with extended family, and the misunderstanding of the developmental stages of a child's life have created a pattern in the last generation or two of overprotecting and isolating children from the reality of death.

In a sense, hospice care is a return to village culture of the past, when the family was the context of all significant experiences, neighbors cared for neighbors and death was a reality of life in the home. Children were as much a part of the communal experience of village culture as adults.

Children need to participate *as children* in the hospice situation. Their questions need to be answered thoughtfully and carefully. Their contacts with the dying patient need to be maintained. The situation needs to be kept as natural and normal as possible for the child. They need sizable additional support to compensate for the inevitable reduction of attention.

Hospice workers can describe instance after instance when both children and the patient have had very good shared experiences. In one situation, a child continued relating to a dying grandparent by bringing every day a drawing of an activity or event from that day. Their conversations became a very important part of their relationship. In another family, when the death occurred early in the morning the family decided to delay the removal of the body until the children awoke, because they had been so positively involved with the patient. They talked about the death and said an appropriate good-bye before the body was taken from the home. To an unenlightened observer such instances might seem unduly morbid, but there is a growing body of evidence that such willing involvement is a positive contribution to effective mourning.[6]

Pastoral Care to Children in the Family

If the family has been part of the life of the church, the pastor is acquainted with both the parents and the children. In the pastoral care given in the hospice situation which involves children, the caregiver has a responsibility to *every member* of the family.

Most of the pastors interviewed could cite occasions when parents turned to them for help in interpreting to a child what was happening. Many pastors offered literature dealing with children and death. That is a helpful resource, but we need constantly to be reminded that literature should be a supplement to relationship. The parents' or the pastor's willingness to talk with, not to instruct, a child is even more important than having all the right information. Literature frequently is not a helpful resource, as some pastors with whom this was discussed pointed out, because the sheer busyness of many home care situations does not permit a lot of reading on the part of parents.

The pastoral caregiver's counsel to parents who seek help should make two points: Permit children to be involved and answer questions as simply and directly as possible. Hospice feels a special responsibility to help children relate meaningfully to the dying patient and to assist them with grieving after death occurs. Family closeness and solidarity are tremendously important in this. Children need to be included rather than isolated. Of course, children should never be forced into involvement. Reluctance probably means that they are responding to some adult input that is creating anxiety for them. Parents, hospice caregivers, and the pastor can be helpful in presenting attitudes which neutralize such negative input without any coercion.

Death is a mystery for everyone, not only children. Every person has developed his or her own mythic or symbolic answers to questions about death and its consequences. One is often tempted to use these adult answers to respond to the questions of children about death. Young children, under the age of nine or ten, are not capable of understanding the abstractions that are involved in most adult answers. They may be able to repeat the words but they do not have the mental ability to find meaning in those abstractions.

The questions that children ask should be heard as children's questions, not adult philosophical or theological inquiries. The most helpful answers for their questions are simple, factual, experiential; they should describe what happens when a person dies and what we experience in terms of not having that person present with us any longer.

When a patient died during the night, a six-year-old son's question was, "What happened to Daddy?" During the illness the child had spent some quality time with both father and mother. In answer to his question his mother said, "You know that Daddy was very sick. His body just wasn't working any more and couldn't be fixed. So last night he died. That makes us all very sad. We'll miss having him here with us." This was followed by assurances that the little boy was very much loved and that his mother and grandparents would always take care of him. As further questions were asked, they were answered in the same simple, direct way, rather than with talk about going to heaven or living with Jesus.

Of course, any thoughtful parent or pastor is well aware of these points, but in the anxiety and the pressure of the situation of terminal illness and death, and impelled by their own need for answers, they may take the easier route of providing conventional adult answers.

Often parents are concerned that their own strong emotions in this situation will have adverse effects on their children. They do not want their own emotional distress to further destabilize the family situation. Rather than isolating their children or suppressing their own feelings, the pastor may be able to encourage parents to use their feelings as channels for developing empathy with their children—sharing feelings openly, discussing how they stand with each other in times of distress and pain. Shared feeling which can be talked about can tie children into the family rather than being a destabilizing influence.

Everyone, including the pastor, should be doing everything possible to normalize the situation for children. Of course, this is relative. A family disrupted by terminal illness can hardly be thought of as living normally. But their experience can be characterized as normal for a family that is coping with the imminent death of one of its members. Normality or health under those circumstances includes a great deal of intentional caring, openness, willingness to share feeling, mutual understanding, and acceptance of individual responses. The pastor may be in a position to model this kind of normalcy for parents.

When the dying patient is a parent, there is often a concern for how the child will cope with the loss after death has occurred. Pastors have been able to be helpful by assuring the parent that they will spend time with the child after the death. In order for this to be a meaningful promise the pastor will have to relate warmly with the child during the period of illness.

One pastor, in describing his pastoral care for children following a death, said that he includes a children's story in the funeral. Such stories deal with empathy, support, and enduring love in the face of death. They speak to the needs of the child for stability and security, rather than attempting to translate adult interpretations of death into childish terms.

The pastor also needs to ensure that the child from a home where there is terminal illness, or from a home where a death has occurred, is supported in the church school setting. Teacher training should include this possibility. Teachers of all grades should be encouraged to respond candidly to the child and his or her peers. Stories should be used to encourage discussion. Questions should be encouraged and answered sensitively. The community of the church can have meaning at any age level.

When the Dying Patient Is a Child

Most hospices, for purely demographic reasons, rarely have a child as a patient. For the same reason most parishes do not have frequent contact with terminally ill children. So there has not been great attention given to pastoral care in such situations.

In fact, there are some who have said that pastoral care is not really effective or necessary for children. If people approach pastoral care of the terminally ill from a rationalistic perspective that emphasizes the need for proper understanding of what is taking place, obviously a child would be incapable of such theological reflection. Or if the aim of pastoral care for the dying is to secure an act of contrition to assure them of heaven, then, as someone has said, "Dying children [will not be] offered pastoral care because people think they are going to heaven anyway."

Children live very much in the present tense, so pastoral care will focus on present experience, the here and now. A child patient will be encouraged to talk about his or her perceptions of what is going on. Drawing and playing with toys can sometimes be more effective communication tools than language.

Telling stories that relate to the child's present situation, the love and care and support that are available, can be very helpful.

Special attention in such a situation must often be paid to the anger felt by parents, siblings, and grandparents. The death of a child seems so unfair. It is much more difficult to see it as a natural process, because aging is not a factor. The psychological and theological defenses that are frequently erected against the threat of mortality seem somewhat empty when applied to the situation of a dying child. One cannot say, "He lived a long, full life," or, "It is a blessing that rest has come."

Ministering to the terminally ill child is a reminder of how often we limit pastoral care to the cognitive and rational. Too often pastors assume that the primary pastoral function is to clarify a person's thinking or to instruct them in church doctrines. Ministering to children helps us see that pastoral care does not hinge merely on understanding a situation or reflecting theologically upon it. Pastoral care is making a person feel cared for: by relating, by making contact with a person at a feeling level. The helpful pastor will spend time with a child, playing, sharing experiences and feelings, and giving full attention to what this child is doing and saying. Effective pastoral care will respond sensitively to the emotional responses to what is being experienced at the time by a person of any age.

Summary

Pastoral care, even though it may be focused on the particular needs of a given individual, always has to be responsive to the context in which that person is living, and in the case of hospice, dying. It is not simply a matter of being aware of the context, but also of responding to that context with caring and a sense of pastoral responsibility to the entire family, not only the dying patient.

NOTES

1. David S. Greer and Vincent Mor, "How Medicare Is Altering the Hospice Movement," *Hastings Center Report* 15, no. 5 (Oct. 1985): 5-9.

2. John Hinton, *Dying* (Baltimore: Penguin Books, 1967), p. 120.

3. Liston O. Mills, "Issues for Clergy in the Care of the Dying and the Bereaved," in *Dying and Death,* ed. David Barton (Baltimore: Williams & Wilkins, 1977), p. 207.

4. Kenneth B. Wentzel, *To Those Who Need It Most, Hospice Means Hope* (Boston: Charles River Books, 1981), p. 71.

5. Edward F. Dobihal, Jr., and Charles William Stewart, *When a Friend Is Dying* (Nashville: Abingdon Press, 1984), pp. 74-75.

6. See Rudolf Toch, "Bereavement: A Pediatric View," in *Death and Ministry,* ed. J. Donald Bane et al. (New York: Seabury Press, 1975), pp. 120-25.

CHAPTER 7

CONTROL ISSUES

Any helping relationship involves control issues. A person has to be willing to be helped, to make himself or herself sufficiently vulnerable to indicate a need. Another person has to be willing to help, to limit herself or himself by accepting responsibility to care for another. In each instance, a person gives over some control of his or her life to another individual; this is true even in the most positive helping relationships.

The hospice caregiver is willing to recognize the extent to which terminally ill patients and families feel that they have very little power. Every little bit of control they can exercise is of tremendous value to their diminished sense of self. So the helper is willing to give up the rewards her or his own ego gets from having control in favor of supporting the right of patients and families to maintain as much control as possible.

Furthermore, given the imperfections of human relationships, there is always the possibility that such giving and taking of control will move toward the excesses of manipulation, beyond the need for help or the need to help. People become manipulative when they feel that they cannot exercise power legitimately.

How does one distinguish between expression of a

legitimate need and a manipulative desire to control? Consider some examples of manipulative behavior: One patient called his physician every few days to ask for a home visit, although his condition was not changing. In spite of his inability to describe any changes or intensification of symptoms, he kept asking the doctor to come. Another patient kept telling her family that she was in the act of dying, even though there was no clinical evidence to indicate this. She repeatedly called the hospice office by day and the on-call nurse by night to state that she was dying. In another instance, every time the patient complained of her symptoms, her husband began to complain of severe chest pain for which no clinical cause could be found. Manipulative behavior is suggested when the need that motivates the request of the person for help is quite different from the need for which relief is being overtly sought.

The interdisciplinary hospice team usually detects a patient's manipulative behavior because everyone is being manipulated. The temptation is to respond with anger or resistance. However, a manipulative person is not helped by others' giving in to the manipulation. Because the individual is motivated by a desire for secondary gain, such as to enhance the self-image by controlling others, the most constructive help is given by talking openly about what is going on. In the context of caring for the manipulative person and his or her needs for positive relationships, the person may be helped to pursue the goals of constructive decision making rather than simply controlling other people.

Self-determination and Decision Making

Participation, as has been pointed out, is a fundamental element in the hospice philosophy. Many terminally ill persons and their families feel overwhelmed by their situations, physically, emotionally, and spiritually. There seems to be little that they can do to stop the ravages of the disease: growing weakness, immobility, loss of control over body functions. They struggle to maintain balance as they are faced with a loss that will disrupt virtually every dimension of their lives. There are times when they feel abandoned and insecure.

In an effort to help people deal with this growing sense of impotence, hospice tries to empower them in those areas in which they *can* exercise some meaningful control. They are encouraged to verbalize their wishes and expectations. Wherever possible, hospice will support them in exercising their freedom of choice. Major exceptions would be if the wishes of one patient or family member seriously disadvantaged another, or if the decision were obviously not contributing to the well-being of the patient and family. Then further discussion would be encouraged.

This represents a departure from standard medical practice, in which the patient gives over the power of decision making to the medical authorities. There are undoubtedly times in the treatment of a disease when such delegation of power is very much justified, although current concern with informed consent is fostering much more sharing of information and options. But in the situation of terminality, different considerations may be involved. The input of the physician is certainly appropriate, but it is no longer the only factor in decision making.

Dobihal and Stewart suggest that control is given by letting patients express their wants and needs.

> "Mrs. _____, what is it you want?" is a question often asked by hospice physicians or nurses or clergy as care is given to the terminally ill. The care-giver listens carefully for the answer and helps patients sort through a number of answers, which can then be addressed in care. . . .

139

It is extremely important for pastoral care-givers to ask this question, "What is it you want?" since unless the ill person is in a hospice program, nobody else may be asking it. It is seldom asked in the hospital setting. There it is assumed that the patient came to be cured, to solve a particular physical problem, and tests and treatments begin on that assumption. It's hard to say and be heard, "I want to be made more comfortable and to be allowed to die in some peace."[1]

Knowledge is power. If it assumed that persons have the right to control their own destinies, the more they know of their situations, the better they can exercise that control. If they are expected to allow others to make their decisions for them, they have no need to know.

In our time, the focus on human rights has come to include the right to know and the corresponding freedom to decide. New and important attention in health care has recently been given to the ethical issue of informed consent. Patients need to know the nature of their situations, the options open to them, and the risks associated with each option. This contemporary concern acknowledges the right to have control over one's own life.

Hospice, with its dedication to openness, believes knowledge contributes to the empowerment of patients and families. The assumption is that people are capable of understanding and assessing their situations and of making sound decisions about how their remaining days will be lived.

Unwillingness to talk with patients about their situations has often been motivated by a desire to protect people from reality. It assumes that patients do not have the emotional stamina to honestly confront their conditions or that there is no need for them to know, since all meaningful decisions will be made for them anyway.

The result of such condescension was that patients' egos were depleted by feelings of powerlessness, and that families were denied the opportunity to share with one another the profound experiences of loving separation. Hospice care is focused on avoiding such unproductive outcomes and on enabling people to deal openly and honestly with the reality of their situations.

So far, power and control issues have been discussed as if patients and families were a monolithic unit. This is not always the case. Control issues may arise between the patient and members of his or her family. Generally, it is assumed that the interests of the patient should have pre-eminent importance. Davidson says: "In the hospice setting, dying persons have purposes and goals, even *in extremis,* which are their own goals, independent of those of family, neighbors, or caregivers. These goals need no justification in terms of social utility. . . . The personal space of the dying is radically 'theirs.' "[2] Our society generally values the wishes of a dying person above all others. The pastoral caregiver, however, will have to be alert for those situations in which the exceptional needs of a family member need to be considered. If openness is really part of the picture, such "conflicts of interest" can be explored, mutual understanding achieved, and decisions made which take into account the diversity of needs. Control that is yielded voluntarily is quite different from power that is denied or withdrawn.

Areas in Which Patient and Family Participation Are Desired

Not all of the areas in which patients and families need to establish some control will be given the same attention here. This is not intended to indicate that some are unimportant. Some of the areas are dealt with in more detail in other chapters and are only included here to show the range of areas in which many hospice patients feel the need for some control.

One pastoral caregiver said, "Patients experience life out of control, so they really feel need for structure." An attempt is made to bring some order out of the chaotic circumstances of life at this point. This can only be done if persons feel that they have some power to regulate the elements of daily living.

In chapter 4 we discussed pain control. Most pain control measures make a patient dependent on the help of some other person to prescribe, provide, and administer medication. Even here, the patient is not passive in that process but is clearly aware that her or his comfort level is one of the determining factors in planning pain control. Control of pain is balanced with some other factors of the patient's and family's needs and wishes, for example, the desire for the lucidity that makes relationships possible. Often patients will opt for limited discomfort and alertness. Although very often both goals can be achieved simultaneously through careful regulation of the medication, if a choice is necessary, the patient's wishes need to be carefully considered.

Another area in which hospice patients want control is over the style of their dying: heroic or palliative treatment, at home or as an in-patient, relating to others or withdrawn, actively involved or passive. The freedom of the patient to die his or her own death, to approach death at whatever depth he or she wishes, is a right granted by hospice. The effectiveness of hospice in enabling this exercise of freedom was indicated in the words of one of the pastors interviewed: "I firmly believe that the time of death is more controlled by the patient at home than in the hospital. Perhaps that is why the predictions of time remaining made by the doctor in the hospital often are so far off when the patient returns home." This may be somewhat generalized, but hospice staffs can point to numerous occasions when it seemed quite apparent that the act of dying was volitional. Patients communicate that they sense the fittingness of a particular moment to die. Without despair, without struggle, they simply lean back and die. This may be the ultimate in maintaining control of one's dying.

Hospice sees that it has something to offer only to those who choose to forgo heroic measures and die with dignity. It fully acknowledges the validity of persons making other decisions, though. Some may elect aggressive treatment, because they have a strong hope that they will recover from their illness. Some may choose to use every tool of medical technology as an act of social responsibility, offering themselves as experimental subjects so that in future others may be assured help. Hospice makes no judgment of right or wrong about these choices, affirming the right of individuals to decide. The making of a free and responsible decision, whatever it might be, is the good that is pursued.

Controlling one's style of dying is somewhat related to where one chooses to live out the final weeks of life. In standard hospital practice, the entire system is based on caregivers being in control. Location, activity, diet, schedule, visitation, attire, and treatments are all regulated by the caregivers, and the patient is expected to acquiesce. Institutional realities make this quite understandable. It would be very difficult to provide care for several hundred patients under one roof without a regulating system.

Hospice care, in either in-patient or home settings, is much more relaxed. From a time-management perspective, hospice seems inefficient. Nurses will not only perform their nursing tasks but will spend a good bit of time talking with the patient and family. Doing something to or for the patient is replaced by doing something with the patient. The patient's and the family's direct, active involvement is encouraged and utilized in care.

Pastoral care is no exception to this approach. The pastor who is committed to caregiving for hospice patients has to make appropriate adjustments to standard approaches. Visits are necessarily time-consuming, because it is important for parishioners to talk through what they are experiencing and how they are understanding it in light of their faith and their commitments.

Parishioners often have the sense that they are facing a profound experience for which they want to prepare themselves spiritually. Some want to feel forgiveness for their sins, some want to make a final commitment of their lives, still others want to try to see their dying in the context of their faith. Some may want to work these issues through by themselves, or may give evidence that they are coping well.

Patients and families should have a significant part in shaping the pastoral relationship. This participation helps pastors learn from hospice that there is no standard or normative way to prepare for one's death. Simplistic, mechanical formulas are not appropriate answers, because they do not take sufficient account of individual needs. Rituals are valuable, but to have fuller meaning their administration needs to be accompanied by a lot of conversation about what that ritual means to the patient and family. One pastor described offering to the patient a brief service of commendation of the dying, very shortly before death. The family was deeply appreciative, because for them it was a way of releasing their loved one and giving "permission" for her to die.

Most pastors probably have not experienced a parishioner who exercised sufficient control of the pastoral relationship to decline a pastoral conversation. Conventions of courtesy more often prevent parishioners from maintaining control. It is quite in keeping with the basic pattern of hospice care for a person to feel free to say, "Thank you, but I don't need you today," or, "Call first to see if I'm feeling up to a visit." This is not necessarily a limitation on pastoral care. It is an affirmation of the freedom of the parishioner to be in control, which is health giving. It also recognizes that without readiness on the part of the parishioner, pastoral care may well be perfunctory.

Pastors, like other hospice caregivers, need to recognize that self-limitation is one of the channels for empowerment of others. To think that someone needs our help strokes our egos, and it is difficult to give over the control that is experienced in being helpful. Yet for some this relinquishment may be the ultimate pastoral service.

Sometimes the patient's desire for control involves a conflict between individual needs and church rules. A pastor was requested to visit a hospice patient who had once been a member of the pastor's particular congregation. In the course of the visit the patient asked to receive the eucharist when the pastor came again. The pastor explained that this was not possible until the patient was again a member of the church. This was interpreted as a rejection by the patient, who became very upset. However, it was of such importance to him that after a few days he yielded and was taken into the church by re-profession of faith, and then received communion.

When this case was described to a number of the pastors interviewed, there was recognition of the "theological correctness" of the approach while at the same time dissatisfaction with the legalistic way in which the patient was handled. The interviewed pastors stated that care for the person should be put before ecclesiastical rules. One stated, "I want to err on the side of the gospel. I want to give *too* much." Another said, "I want to err on the side of love." Generally, the pastors wanted to avoid creating any sense of rejection in the patient.

One pastor described her way of dealing with requests for pastoral service that call for a bending of church rules. She explains to the patient or family, "Normally, I wouldn't do it this way, but I will do it." Then they talk, not about the substance of the rules, but of what this request means to the patient.

Hospice staffs, with their commitment to advocacy for the patient, are naturally distressed by situations in which patients feel rejected because of a pastor's singular devotion to church rules. They need to know which pastors have such limitations and to be aware of the specific religious customs and practices of various churches, to avoid disruptive situations.

Control Issues

The need for control extends to at least four important dimensions of the patient's life: space, self, relationship, and time.

1. Issues of Space

A few years ago an interesting study of animals introduced the notion of "territoriality." We all share the sense of needing personal space over which we have a sizable measure of control.

In the hospice situation, this need for control over space has an influence on decisions about where the patient wants to be cared for and where he or she wants to die. Although this is partly a matter of sentiment, it also is a way of expressing territoriality. It has already been pointed out how some settings enable more personal control than others. Only when special levels of care are needed or when care is not available in the home will patients choose to trade off control of personal space for the care they require. That decision itself, provided it is made by and not for the patient, is an exercise of control over space.

2. Issues of Self—My Body

Our bodies are part of our perception of ourselves. The body changes of terminal illness, all of which are losses, bring along an altered picture of the self as painful, wasted, dysfunctional, diminished. There is not much, beside pain control, that can be done to reverse the loss of body function, but caregiving can focus on keeping these losses from reducing the patient's efforts to maintain a measure of control over his or her life. Dobihal and Stewart show how this becomes a control issue:

> A primary need of the terminally ill—a need that is partly emotional, as well as social and spiritual—is to maintain some feeling of control over one's life. When the body is sick we are aware of it, our total self is sick, we are out of control. We need to regain some of that sense of control, and that can happen if it is clear that our wishes, our wants, our ability to participate in decisions about our life are being respected.[3]

Some of the most common questions regarding control of one's body are, Should additional surgery be attempted even though it promises to extend life only a little longer? Should repeated blood transfusions be administered to provide temporary strength to the patient? Should antibiotics be used to treat pneumonia in a terminal cancer patient? One patient expressed it by saying to his pastor, "I want to be treated like a well person until the time when I'm really sick." At first the pastor thought this was denial, but when they talked about it further, the patient was really saying that he wanted to maintain control over the decisions that were being made about continuing chemotherapy. The pastor, along with others of the hospice staff, can help by being a strong patient advocate. Patients need to be asked repeatedly, "What do *you* want?" and then supported in making those wishes into reality. Pastors have the opportunity to ask the question in another form. Before praying with a patient it is quite appropriate to ask, "What would you like to pray for?" Pastoral conversations about the patient's future expectations, when communicated to hospice staff, can set directions for guiding future care in accordance with the patient's wishes.

3. Issues of Relationship

Patients have every right to control who they wish to have near during the remainder of their lives. Some patients want to be surrounded with many relatives and friends. One hospice patient functioned as a hostess, daily entertaining groups of old friends at her bedside with conversation and refreshments. It was important to her to make the most of her days in the company of her family and friends.

Sometimes earlier fractures in a family get woven into the pattern of controlling relationships. Estrangements carry over into the period of terminality. The patient may wish for reconciliation with an alienated family member, or, conversely, the patient may not want to see the estranged. While maintaining the patient's right to control relationships, pastoral caregivers can help people talk about the alienation and sort out their reasons for feeling as they do. No pressure is exerted to force reconciliation, but often having someone with whom deep hurts from the past can be shared removes the need to keep acting out these injuries through punitive, isolating behavior.

4. Issues of Time

Because not much attention has been given in preceding chapters to the issue of controlling time, it will receive fuller treatment here than the three control issues just discussed. For the terminally ill person, all three dimensions of time have special meaning: The present carries with it a sense of urgency; the past is repeatedly assessed; the future raises questions of hope.

Time itself cannot be controlled; it marches inexorably on quite independent of our wishes. But the way time is used is subject to our control and is an issue for many hospice patients. Consider the name of a highly effective self-help group for cancer patients: "Make Today Count."

Unlike the past and the future, which have sizable private dimensions—my memories, my hopes—*present time* is a shared experience. Other people are experiencing the same moment in time simultaneously. So efforts to control the use of present time often involve efforts to control the use of the time by others. Patients may wish to fill present time only with quality experiences. One patient gave his wife a list of friends he wanted to visit him regularly and those with whom he wanted only casual and less frequent contact. The significant variable was the willingness of the friends to acknowledge his situation. He had little time for those who acted like nothing profound was going on in his life; he wanted to share his present moments with those who knew how precious those were for him. The hospice environment is often a signal to friends that it is all right to talk openly with the patient about his or her situation, rather than filling the time with innocuous diversionary conversation.

Many hospice patients want time to be used in ways that will apparently protract the present; they want a slower pace of life. Like members of the hospice staff, the pastoral caregiver will communicate an understanding of this by taking time to listen in the context of unhurried visits. It is not simply a matter of the length of time, but of the ways in which the time is used to deal with the patient's agenda.

It is not unusual to detect a sense of urgency in the

patient's requests. Some of the pastors interviewed had sensed in patients a desire for immediate gratification. One described a patient who became very upset when a pastor did not respond quickly to a request for a visit, but postponed it several times due to other plans.

A pastor might easily become annoyed at such apparently manipulative behavior, unless there was an understanding of the urgency experienced by the patient. One could interpret such demands for immediate gratification as being caused by the infantile regression sometimes associated with serious illness. Or it could be due to the sense of having so little time left to live. Or it could be the acting out of a need to regulate a life that feels out of control. In any instance, the sensitive pastor will respond in ways that take the urgency seriously.

The need to control time is also apparent in the pronounced desire of some patients for regularity. A number of the pastors contacted confirmed that some hospice patients want pastoral visits to be on a regular schedule. This may be traceable in part to a pattern of closely scheduled living that was part of the patient's life-style prior to the illness. But for many hospice patients pain medication is closely scheduled and this regularity carries over into the rest of their day. Their schedule is a way of controlling time.

Pastors adopt a variety of ways of responding to these patient wishes. One pastor said, "People know that I can be reached at any time and that I will come. Once people know that you care enough to respond quickly, they relax. Actually, demands may be a way of testing if you care." Several pastors visit by appointment, phoning in advance of the visit. They pointed out that they had to be scrupulously faithful to the commitment to visit at an appointed time. In the rare exceptions where appointments had to be changed, they phoned the patient or family and arranged a new time as soon as possible. A number of pastoral caregivers negotiated a visiting pattern with hospice patients, committing themselves to visit weekly, or two or three times a week, often at a pre-determined time. They found that patients were much more satisfied with such a scheduled pattern than they were with random visits. There is comfort in knowing, when life seems to be shifting around under you, that some meaningful events can be counted on to occur with regularity.

One of the links between the present and *the past* is the sense of having to make up for lost time. Some patients become aware of shortcomings in their past living and use the present moments to try to make up for those deficiencies.

As human beings, we are aware of living in a historical process and having personal histories linking us to our past. Memories are a part of our everyday experience. Terminality, which brings on a sense of the preciousness of time, causes life to be reviewed from the special perspective of awareness that it is drawing to a close. A great deal of reminiscing is done—reviewing past happiness, talking about past failures and disappointments, trying to see patterns of meaning in the life that has been lived to this point.

Some terminally ill persons quite literally try to recapitulate parts of their pasts. They want to revisit places that have been important locales in their lives. They want to experience some events one last time. They want to visit with persons who have shared particular experiences with them. Others will recapitulate mentally, rehearsing their memories.

Davidson describes this process very helpfully, in terms of the experience of mourners.

When mourners talk about themselves, to reminisce, particularly about their relationships with the deceased, they are engaging in a ritual process as old as mankind. They are calling up from the unconscious past those cues which previously oriented them to reorder the seeming chaos of the present. Robert Butler calls this process 'life review' while anthropologists of religion term it the telling of myths.[4]

But when we recall that hospice patients are mourning in anticipation of their approaching deaths, the relevance of this description for the dying person's review of his or her own past becomes readily apparent.

Memories of the past can be pleasant or unpleasant, comforting or disruptive, good or bad. The pastoral caregiver can assist this life review process by being a willing listener to the rehearsal of the past. The priceless quality of good memories can be acknowledged.

But the pastor has an even more important function in helping people to process the bad memories. The traditional priestly role of confessor, manifested either through formal ritual or casual pastoral conversation, provides a context for the pastor to join the patient in a review of his or her life. This is not to suggest a compulsive, scrupulous search for every unresolved issue, but rather that the pastor will be open to talk about any part of the patient's past that the patient wishes to bring up. The past cannot be changed; it is simply there. But one's response to the past can be shaped and reshaped. There can be healing, as new and positive responses emerge, redeeming the past.

The personal agendas of almost all hospice patients contain elements of unfinished business, which the pastor can help resolve in two ways. One is by being willing to talk about all of them, sorting out those things which can be changed and acknowledging those things which cannot. The other pastoral function is to free the patient from scrupulosity, the feeling that every sin has to be confessed, every wrong righted, every loose end tied up. The pastoral message is that of grace: The healing of the wounds of the past is not brought about solely by our actions of restitution but by loving acceptance. In the mode of Tillich's "courage to be," we experience acceptance even though we acknowledge the unacceptability of our past.

The link between the present moment and *the future* is hope, the expectation that the road we travel goes on and on. When terminal illness draws the horizon in very close, the need for hope becomes all the more pronounced. We have already discussed hope in some detail in chapter 5 and look at it here as it offers a way to feel some control over one's future.

Daily life for every person is filled with short-term and long-term hopes. These are defined by the goals that dot all our hours and days. All of our activity is focused on accomplishing some kind of goal: going from here to there, finishing this task, meeting this person. There are longer range goals as well: to finish college, to establish a home, to advance one's career. And there are goals of ultimate proportions: to live a good life, to endure beyond illness and death. Hope draws us on with the possibility of reaching or approximating these goals of various proportion. We cannot move forward from this present moment without some sense of hope to draw us into the future.

Hope, like the future, by its very nature requires a leap of faith. It is prepared to take the risk that the hope will not be fulfilled. The person who has hope has the courage to trust that a goal can be reached, without feeling that he or she must single-handedly bring hope into actuality.

Robert Lifton has noted five ways in which people who are dying or grieving express hope for the future.[5] Some hope in terms of biological immortality: living on after death through one's children and thus continuing to participate in the genetic pool. Others frame their hope in the form of social immortality, in which the creativity of one's life endures in contributions that have been made to the lives of others. Still others interpret their hope for the future as the ongoingness of the natural process. One's life may end, but the process of which one has been a part lives on. Yet another way of portraying hope is to think of dying as an experience of ecstasy, of absorption into a transcendental reality. Finally, there is the theological view expressed in Judeo-Christian imagery as life after death, in which personal existence continues or is restored in a spiritual life beyond death.

It is understandable that persons cling very hard to their own expressions of hope for the future beyond death. The need to somehow overcome death is very strong, as is the need to control the future. So people are heavily invested in whatever form their hope is expressed and assume that their way is true. They tend to be very defensive of that interpretation, which is part of their way of controlling the future.

Actually, what a person thinks or believes is only a personal reflection, not the substance of truth. Just by thinking something, we do not make it true. In a sense, any of the five ways in which Lifton describes hope for overcoming death could be true. One selects from them the way that is most personally meaningful and helpful, to shape one's perception of the future.

Expressing hope is a creative way of adapting to one's perception of the future. For the hospice patient, the immediate future is foreshortened. Five- or ten-year plans are irrelevant. So the person seeks meaning by positing a future beyond the experience of death and expresses that hope in ways that are personally meaningful. The patient does not stay fixated on the past to slow down the passage of time, but by engaging the future with courage lives out the remaining days hopefully.

Summary

Hospice is dedicated to empowering people to be actively involved in their dying. This means that patients and their families are participants, not observers. Hospice encourages people to leave the passivity to which they may have become accustomed in extended illness and to take control of important dimensions of their lives and deaths. This requires special attitudes on the part of caregivers, because so often caregiving ends up trying to control the attitudes and behaviors of those who are helped. Pastoral care can be a meaningful part of the empowerment of patients and families.

NOTES

1. Edward F. Dobihal, Jr., and Charles William Stewart, *When a Friend Is Dying* (Nashville: Abingdon Press, 1984), pp. 60-61.
2. Glen W. Davidson, *The Hospice: Development and Administration*, 2nd ed. (Washington: Hemisphere Publishing Corp., 1985), p. 165.
3. Dobihal and Stewart, *When a Friend Is Dying*, p. 20.
4. Davidson, *The Hospice*, p. 146.
5. Robert Jay Lifton, "The Politics of Immortality," *Psychology Today* (Nov. 1970): 70ff.

CHAPTER 8

THE BLEND OF PROFESSIONAL
AND LAY CAREGIVERS

One of the unique dimensions of hospice is the way in which professional and lay caregivers relate in the hospice team. Using volunteers is nothing new, but to view them as peers is an innovation. Hospitals, for example, are full of pink ladies, gray ladies, and candy-stripers, but the tasks they perform are largely menial and superficial: transporting patients, delivering flowers and mail, staffing information desks. These are all helpful tasks, to be sure, but they are only tangentially related to actual patient care, which is totally provided by professionals.

Lay Involvement in Hospice

In hospice, lay volunteers are very much a part of the program. In fact, having a corps of trained lay volunteers is a requirement of hospice standards. Insurers, quite naturally, are interested in the cost savings accomplished by having some services provided by unpaid volunteers. Supporters of the hospice philosophy see much broader values in participation of lay caregivers, values which also have relevance in the life of the church.

Most hospices in the United States had their beginnings in the interest and action of a group of volunteer community leaders. Many hospices, unless founded by an existing health care institution, started with unpaid professional staff as well. But a vital component was the carefully selected and trained group of lay volunteers who related meaningfully to patients *alongside* staff members with professional training and competence.

The function of lay volunteers was to provide direct patient service, which in the holistic understanding of hospice meant something other than regulating and administering medication, changing dressings, and inserting catheters. Patients and families also needed emotional support, companionship in their crisis, someone to provide respite from their heavy burdens of care.

Probably the simplest definition of a lay volunteer in the hospice program is a person with special competence in dealing with approaching death openly and empathically, who becomes a friend to patients. Though most patients and families have friends, some of whose social conditioning to be evasive or fearful in the presence of the dying makes them less than helpful in accomplishing the goals of hospice care.

Lay volunteers have to understand and be willing to function in accord with the hospice philosophy of holism, the right of patients to participation and self-determination, and openness. They must be able to effectively model such attitudes for patients and their families.

Most hospices discovered a huge community need for their services. The staffs of many community-based hospices, which at the beginning were largely volunteer, were quickly overloaded by requests for both professional and lay assistance. These hospices were immediately faced with the choice of remaining small and denying services to some patients and families or growing to meet the need by engaging paid professional staff to work along with unpaid volunteers.

A recent issue of the *Hastings Center Report* dealt with the changes that are occurring with the professionalization of hospices.[1] The report sees a danger that the enthusiasm and ideological fervor for the hospice concept may be lost, as volunteer community leadership is replaced by professional hospice administrators and staffs. The cautions of this article are appropriate. One measure of the continued support of the hospice philosophy will be the continued meaningful inclusion of lay volunteers as members of the hospice team.

The Value of a Blend of Professional and Lay Caregivers

Hospice, while recognizing the value of very good professional medical and nursing care, also acknowledges the equivalent contribution of simple human caring offered by non-professionals. A volunteer who sits regularly with the patient or family to talk, who spends time with children in the home, who provides the family with some break-time to get out of the house for errands or for respite, who becomes a friend, provides a great deal of care. The recognition that both professional and lay persons share with equal effectiveness in the care of the patient and family confirms the contributions made by each group.

Blending lay persons and professionals in a team widens the perspective of all caregivers. The contributions of lay volunteers help professionals see the value of simple caring. All help does not come through the exercise of professional training and skills. The poise of a friendly volunteer may be as helpful in coping with approaching death as skilled prescription and administration of pain medication. There have been instances when the empathic attitudes of lay volunteers have helped to moderate the stoic toughness in which many professionals have been trained.

Likewise, lay volunteers can see the value of the special competencies of the professional staff: the knowledge that enables pain control, the skill of nurses in solving some of the difficult problems of caring for the patient, the social worker's knowledge of community resources for responding to special problems, the effectiveness of the pastor in helping people find meaning in their pain and loss.

The need for communication in the hospice team requires that professional jargon, which is essentially in-group language, be put aside for a more inclusive means of communication. This opens the way to better communication with the patient and family. There is less temptation to pretension or to obfuscation. The fulfillment of the need to know, which is so much a part of the hospice approach, is supported by the more understandable language encouraged by the conversation of lay and professional caregivers.

Since perfection evades humankind, it is understandable that some problems might also grow out of the blending of professional and lay caregiving. Occasionally a staff member is so imbued with belief in the superiority of professional training that there is arrogant disregard for the innate skills of the lay caregiver. This is an inappropriate attitude in hospice, because it violates the concept of the interdisciplinary team. There is simply no room in hospice for prima donnas.

On the other side, there are occasionally volunteers who stray over into areas of professional practice, exceeding their competence as lay caregivers. Sometimes this is simple pretension to a competence the volunteer does not possess, but more often it is an unthinking response to the request of patient or family. One pastor who works closely with a hospice reported, "Clarity is important. Our volunteers spell out carefully to patients what they can do. But sometimes a volunteer gets sucked into doing more than he or she should do: offering prognoses, commenting on the relative effectiveness of particular medications, counseling in complex situations."

The problems just mentioned are far outweighed by the benefits of the relationship between professional and lay caregivers; and there are some ways of preventing or correcting them. The design of hospice programs, if followed thoughtfully, can do much to avoid the excesses of professional arrogance and lay presumption.

Staff selection is a crucial point in averting problems. Participation in hospice requires the capacity for attitudes of openness, sharing, and humility. The selection process has to give major attention to the motivation of the potential staff member, whether professional or lay.

Non-professionals are usually highly motivated. One would not volunteer for something as difficult as hospice care with only tepid motivation. But strong motivation can be either positive or negative. People may come to a hospice program because they are aware of a profound need and want to make a caring response. They may have been through similar experiences in their own families and want to share some of the benefit they received in coping with their personal losses. But some others are motivated, consciously or unconsciously, by the need to work through their own unresolved grief from a loss, or to proselytize for their faith, or to become a pseudo-practitioner of medicine.

Most hospice programs screen their applicants, train them carefully and provide supervision for their patient care. The goal is to help people to clarify their functions as lay volunteers and to enable them to communicate their functions to patients and families, as well as to fellow caregivers. Clarity is extremely important. A holistic concern does not make a division of labor obsolete. Rather, it establishes a kind of complementarity in which the efforts of a great many persons, both professional and lay, are blended together in service to the patient and family. If it is seen that the efforts of every caregiver are equally valuable and helpful, there is less temptation to step over into areas in which one does not have competence. The efforts of all are equally important for the patient.

Pastoral Caregiving: Lay and Clergy

Pastoral care, as a part of hospice care, involves many of these same issues. The emphasis of the Reformation on the priesthood of all believers, based on scriptural precedents, has provided a strong theological warrant for including the laity in the ministry of the church. But with very few exceptions there still exists a division of labor between professional and lay workers. This distinction is not based on the value of their labors, but is a functional one based on training and the amount of time a person can give to that work.

There are two ways of defining pastoral care: care given by the pastor of a congregation or care that is given with a caring, shepherding approach. In the latter definition, pastoral care can be given by either an ordained or an unordained person. The word "pastoral" describes a function of the church, not just that of a designated leader. The blending of professional and lay ministry is increasingly common in the church.

In addition to the work of the pastor there are three forms which this blending can take in hospice: Members of the church who are relatives or friends of the terminally ill person may provide a form of pastoral care for the patient and family; professional staff or lay volunteers in the hospice program can be pastoral caregivers; or a parish may train selected lay persons for a special lay ministry to the dying. Any or all of these blends may be operative in hospice care.

If pastoral caregiving is defined functionally, anyone who provides such care should be carefully trained and supervised. A very helpful training program is presented in Dobihal and Stewart.[2] Using this approach, the pastor is not seen as the only pastoral caregiver to the dying. Instead he or she assumes responsibility for training lay persons in this function.

In a sense, participation in hospice can support a pastor in working through this important role understanding. One pastor commented: "In a way, the church brought to hospice the caring tools. Now they are being reflected back to the church, helping it to extend pastoral caring."

Surprisingly, however, interviews showed that a fair number of pastors active in hospice did not use lay persons from their congregations as pastoral caregivers to the dying. Evidently, the pastors' learnings from the hospice model have not yet been uniformly transferred to the life of the church.

Values and Problems of Shared Pastoral Caregiving in Hospice

Increased "coverage" of pastoral responsibilities can be one of the advantages of this broader understanding of pastoral care. One pastor who was interviewed said, "Because there are people, trained and attentive to the needs of the patient, it doesn't depend on the minister's being there at the right moment when someone is 'ready to talk.' " This suggests that it is probably best to think of shared pastoral care as supplementing the pastor's caregiving, rather than replacing it.

The pastor who is serious about this kind of lay pastoral caregiving will not only develop a training *and supervising* program in her or his parish, but will also be alert to teaching opportunities in the less structured setting of hospice. The pastor can help people, both professional and lay volunteers, and family members, to see the pastoral implications of what they are doing and their opportunities to share pastorally in some of the reflections of the patient.

A small number of the pastors who were interviewed described problems arising from hospice staff members, either professional or lay, seeking to provide pastoral care. In some instances, these objections grew out of the pastors' theological and ecclesiological understandings of ministry. They defined pastoral ministry in terms of the activity of the ordained pastor.

Others pointed out specific instances in which they felt pastoral caregiving was inadequately provided by untrained lay persons. Some of their comments were, "Hospice staff not trained in pastoral care may blunder. Their theology does not match mine re: heaven, salvation, everlasting life. I am not trained to give shots, yet they feel innately capable of dealing with my field, which took years of study." "Many lay volunteers are not trained, nor do they know what to do with spiritual and religious issues, especially if they are not religious persons themselves."

Where a pastor's conflict with the hospice team's delivery of pastoral care is due to a theological position, the view of ministry must be respected as simply a given. For example, one could not expect a Roman Catholic priest to turn over the responsibility to hear a confession and to grant absolution to a lay person. But where the issue is team members' lack of training and lack of understanding, solutions are available. The pastor can be helpful in pointing up religious needs to members of the hospice team and may become a kind of tutor for staff members and family. The pastor can model sensitivity to spiritual issues, just as hospice staff model behavior and attitudes for the family.

If patients respect a pastor's training and role, understood in the context of their particular church, the pastor does not need to vie with the lay person, for his or her viewpoint will almost automatically receive precedence in the mind of the patient. If the patient does not have regard for that training or role, clerical pressure will only be annoying.

Hospice administrators and supervisors are frequently concerned that professional staff members and lay volunteers not press their own religious views on patients and families. If the right to self-determination, which is so much a part of hospice, is honored by all, including the clergy, people will be supported in working out their own answers to the profound spiritual questions that arise out of their situation. If a hospice caregiver is asked to share her or his own view, that certainly can be done, but it should always be in the context of the right of the patient and family to decide for themselves. Just as manipulative behavior on the part of the patient, which is intended to achieve a secondary gain of domination, is confronted forthrightly, manipulative behavior by a lay pastoral caregiver, which is intended to achieve conversion, is rejected as improper caregiving.

These significant problems can be dealt with by providing information about effective pastoral caregiving and by sensitizing persons to the nature of spiritual needs. The positive result of such training is seen in the experience of a hospice volunteer, who shared in team conference a conversation with a patient. They had been talking about life after death, and the patient had said, "I believe in reincarnation. When someone dies, she enters into this kind of spirit world until it's time to come back in another body." The volunteer reported, "At one time I would have told the person that that was more Hindu than

Christian and that she should believe in resurrection, not reincarnation. But instead I said, 'It really comforts you to think about a person's spirit living on and on. That's important to you right now.' My hospice training really paid off. We had the best talk."

Summary

Hospice and the church are concerned for meeting needs. Both testify that effectiveness in responding to need is not so much a matter of who the helper is as of the sensitivity and caring that the potential helper can provide. There can be effective cross-learning of this reality for both hospice and church.

NOTES

1. Claire Tehan, "Has Success Spoiled Hospice?" *Hastings Center Report* 15, no. 5 (Oct. 1985): 10-13.
2. Edward F. Dobihal, Jr., and Charles William Stewart, *When a Friend Is Dying* (Nashville: Abingdon Press, 1984), pp. 130-59.

CHAPTER 9

BEREAVEMENT AFTERCARE

Dying and grieving are natural processes in hospice. Coping with these two intimately intertwined processes is the central focus of the whole hospice approach.

The Role of Hospice in the Grief Process

It is impossible to be concerned about the dying process without a similar concern about the process of grieving. Hospice understands death in a social as well as a clinical sense. Not only does a life come to an end, but a whole structure of family relationships is lost and has to be rebuilt without the deceased. Things are never the same as they were before the death.

A program of bereavement aftercare is mandated by both the standards of the National Hospice Organization and the Hospice Medicare requirements for certification. From the very beginning of its service, hospice commits itself to maintaining concern for the bereaved family for at least a year following the death of the patient. Many patients are comforted by this commitment because it means that the same caring helpfulness will continue to be extended to their families during the difficult period of adjustment following death.

This commitment to those who survive the death of the patient sets hospice apart from other care delivery systems, which place their sole, or major, focus on the patient. Their perfectly valid institutional self-understanding ends commitment to service when the patient dies. The institutional self-understanding of hospice, on the other hand, requires continuity of service to the grieving family.

Anticipatory Grief

Of course, grief work begins during the patient's dying. Because hospice tries to deal with dying and grieving simultaneously, concern for bereavement is not postponed until death occurs. Hospice mobilizes early on the psychic energy required for grieving because it involves an extended process that begins when the terminal diagnosis is realized and goes on for a considerable time after the death of the patient. Families start by mourning the loss of their hope for a cure and finish by mourning the loss of the patient and celebrating the survival of the family.

The sensitivity of caregivers makes possible the expression of grief and loss even before death. In many ways the hospice team is saying to patients and families that it is perfectly all right, in fact health-giving, to admit your feelings and to show emotion. They are prepared to deal openly with their needs as grieving persons, rather than conforming to the constricting expectations so often advanced by our society.

Hospice caregivers sometimes observe private grieving: The patient is tearful when death is mentioned, the patient's spouse weeps when out of the patient's sight. Part of the function of hospice is to strengthen communication among family members so that the grieving that family members do is actually shared with the dying patient, who also grieves the approaching death. The ability to talk together about this grief, even with tears, can be a very positive experience, easing people into the grief process gradually.

Facilitating patient acceptance of approaching death also appears to have a positive effect on the grieving of family members. There are indications that family grief following the death is less complicated and protracted when the patient has communicated an acceptance of dying.

The Grief Process After Death

After the death of the patient, family members are faced with the task of putting their lives back together without the presence of the deceased. It is not simply a matter of working through the sadness they feel. The swirl of events accompanying the decline of their loved one gradually became a vortex into which their lives were drawn, as they became increasingly involved with the patient's care, spending more and more of their energy on it. Their selfhood has been caught up in this crisis, and when it ends and they no longer have this demanding responsibility, the task of reorienting their lives is sizable.

As Davidson points out:

> From a medical perspective, mourners become *dysfunctional*, which means that day-to-day health needs are not handled as competently as before the loss. From a psychological perspective, mourners become confused, distracted, and preoccupied, so that decision making is difficult. From a theological perspective, mourners become distrustful because they must rethink not only who or what can be trusted, but whether one can trust at all.[1]

Some features of the hospice approach, if they are internalized by family members, can make the grieving process easier. The openness with which death has been acknowledged counteracts the tendency to evade the reality of their loss. The fact that they have been actively involved in the care of the patient, that they have done what they could for the patient, makes them less likely to feel guilt or regret in their grief. The opportunities for closure enable an awareness of the finality of the dissolution of the relationship with the patient and the need for life to go on.

This should not be taken to imply that in every instance family members have an easy, therapeutic grief experience. The fact that persons have been involved with hospice care does not mean that they are automatically imbued with the hospice philosophy. Sometimes their link with hospice is brief, because the patient dies only a few days after admission to the program. Sometimes unproductive patterns for relating to the terminal situation, such as, denial, anger, and anxiety, have developed to such an extent that admission to hospice care cannot reverse them. Sometimes a negative psychological makeup, originating in and reenforced by years of unhealthy relationships, is so strong that participation in hospice care cannot change it completely.

Most hospice families have been helped to develop a greater variety of coping mechanisms. They have been shown that it is helpful to be open in talking about their needs. They have been introduced to a variety of persons and services upon which they can depend for help. They have been taught by hospice that they have legitimate needs for respite and that it is all right to be concerned for themselves and their own needs, even in face of the needs of the dying person. Experience with such coping mechanisms, helpful during the terminal illness, provides guidance for their mourning.

The rights of the family to participation and self-determination extend into the bereavement aftercare program. Some families want to get on with their lives after long disruption. Throughout the long process of caring for the terminally ill patient, they have had to hold their own plans and activities in abeyance. They may opt not to be involved in the aftercare program, either because their need to grieve has been met or because they think that grieving will hold them back from resuming their life-style. Hospice bereavement workers need to help family members assess their needs carefully. It is legitimate to be concerned for too speedy "completion" of grief work, which may later exact a high cost. But just as hospice will accept and work with counterproductive attitudes and actions prior to the death of the patient, it continues to recognize the right of people to decide the course of their own lives. When families do not wish aftercare, hospice continues at most only to offer its services, maintaining periodic contact in ways that do not overwhelm or coerce the family.

Hospice workers sometimes experience this lack of enthusiastic acceptance of aftercare as rejection. They are distressed by the fact that a resource of proven helpfulness is not being used, but there may also be the feeling that the family, now that the pressure of patient care is no longer present, is turning its back on the caring hospice workers. This calls for sensitive examination of the tension between the needs of the helper and those of the person for whom help is intended.

The hospice approach is to help people help themselves. Rather than being passive recipients of service, involvement is fostered wherever possible. Just as one cannot do another person's dying, one cannot do another person's grieving. The help is provided by giving persons resources for working their way through these very difficult and complex processes.

Although each hospice develops its own approach

to bereavement aftercare, some elements are common to all: a closure visit from staff who cared for the patient, attendance at the funeral, periodic contacts by the bereavement coordinator, assignment of a bereavement volunteer to visit and maintain contact with the immediate family.

Even if the hospice staff person, usually the nurse or the volunteer, was present when death occurred, it is a common practice for her or him to pay a visit to the bereaved family a day or so after the death. This visit marks the ending of one phase of hospice care and the beginning of another. It draws to a close the relationship which centered around the patient and focuses now on the needs of the bereaved.

This visit is an opportunity to participate in the sharing of memories of the patient's living and dying, a process necessary to healthy grieving. Nurse and volunteer can support the remembering process. Where hospice care has extended over some weeks or months, hospice staff have very often become very close to the family, and such sharing is very natural.

Many hospices regularly make it possible for a staff member who has been involved with the patient and family to attend the funeral. Recognizing the value of this ritual closure, of the affirmation of those beliefs that sustain in crisis, of the support of gathered friends and relatives, hospice shares in this experience, which symbolizes the holistic approach and communicates sustained support for the family.

It must be recognized that under such circumstances hospice staff who have become friends of the patient and family are mourners as well. They benefit personally from their sharing with the family and from the funeral service.

Many hospices recognize a responsibility to help their staff members with the cumulative grief that comes through dealing with the deaths of a number of patients to whom one has become attached. Not only is there encouragement of informal sharing of feelings between staff persons; often more structured approaches are taken. There are periodic group sessions in which personal grief can be shared and reflected upon, and caring responses given. When bereavement overload occurs, consultation with a psychological counselor or pastoral counselor is arranged, and there is no pressure of persuasion or inflicting of guilt when a staff member chooses to leave the program because of such stress.

Contacts Through the First Year of Bereavement

The selection of a year as the period of hospice commitment suggests to the bereaved that mourning does not go on at the same intensity for year after year. They can hope to make considerable progress toward resolution during that time—with the understanding that no one is demanding that they adhere to a rigid timetable. Following mourners for a year also allows hospice to assist families with the strong feelings that will accompany a year's cycle of birthdays, anniversaries, and holidays.

Special attention is given to those families who have limited resources to support their grieving. If family members indicate that they have a good deal of support from relatives or friends and feel that they are making an effective adjustment to their loss, hospice attention becomes less intense. Or, as one hospice administrator put it, "If there is effective pastoral care by a pastor known to our staff, our hospice does not do as much aftercare."

Ongoing contact with bereaved families takes a number of forms. The hospice staff member, who may be a bereavement counselor or the volunteer who was with the family during the care of the patient, will maintain personal contacts through telephone calls and visits. An effort is made to ensure that contacts are made on a regular schedule, with flexibility to respond to special needs.

Many hospices also have an ongoing support group to which bereaved families are regularly invited. Some hospices use existing groups in the community, while others develop their own programs. Such groups are particularly important in settings where people do not have strong social ties because of urban depersonalization or lack of family. It is often found that bereaved family members do not respond to invitations to such groups until several months after the death. The groups are open-ended. People can join when they are ready and drop out when they no longer feel the need. Persons who continue to experience a need for the group over many months and who are not showing forward movement in their grieving probably will be helped more by personal counseling than by continued membership in the group.

Some hospices also arrange an annual interfaith service memorializing all those who have died during the year. This offers an opportunity for many families who have in their own ways shared an experience to come together supportively and to remember the deceased in the context of a religious ritual.

Pastoral Care of Bereaved Hospice Families

Pastoral care of the bereaved has long been an important part of the ministry of the church and has been a significant focus in the literature of pastoral care and counseling.[2] The particular focus in this volume is on the special dimensions of such pastoral care provided when bereaved parishioners are involved in hospice.

The commitment of hospice to provide bereavement aftercare for a year is a helpful model for pastoral care. Too often pastors have confined pastoral care to a relatively brief period following a death unless persons were showing pathological distress. This is even more common following terminal illness, where it has been assumed that a lot of grieving has been done in anticipation of the death. This has left people to finish their grief work without adequate pastoral care. Some of the best studies that have been made in recent years have indicated that grieving takes time and that there are periods during the first year of bereavement when acute grief returns, as defenses against it prove inadequate.[3]

Pastoral care of the bereaved, whoever provides it, has six functions: to assist people to face the reality of their loss, to support the process of remembering the deceased, to encourage the expression of authentic feelings, to provide a supportive presence, to aid in the reorientation to a new life without the person who has died, and to help in finding a personally satisfying way to give meaning to the death and its consequences.

The resources for grieving that have been accentuated by participation in a hospice program include the highly supported open dealing with death and loss during the illness, the recognition of the connection between anticipatory grief and the grieving that follows death, the modeling of the free expression of feelings and personal needs, the importance of accepting support rather than stoically going it alone, and the strength gained by putting the death into the context of one's faith or value system.

The dying person and family members struggled with the question of how to fit the death into the universe as they understand it, into the ongoing life process, into their understanding of God's purpose. These same questions continue during the period of bereavement. Like a ship at sea, grieving people have to fix their position somehow; they need to know how their experience of loss fits into the pattern that gives meaning to life.

Part of gaining that navigational fix, to continue the metaphor, is to know the course that has already been traveled. The pastoral caregiver will encourage bereaved families to review the ways they struggled to find meaning for what has happened in their lives during the time that they cared for the patient.

Through such recollecting, the mourners engage in the same sort of life review as the terminally ill do, according to Davidson. The meanings that people give to death and its consequences are the endings for the story which they tell. Davidson writes:

> As you first tell your story, you will probably not be able to provide an ending. Some people try. They say things like, "This is God's will," or "It was meant to be." More unfortunate are those mourners who, in trying to tell their story, are given endings by other people who share "words of advice," give "testimony," or respond with clichés. . . .
>
> Telling the story of your loss over and over is more important than having a "right ending," at least for a while. . . .
>
> You will need to tell your story of loss and change again and again in order to get your facts straight, clarify how you are part of the facts, discover how your life has been changed by those facts, and finally to determine how you fit into the arrangements of the universe. Some people refer to these tasks in theological terms as they try to find how, even in their changed world, they fit into God's order.[4]

The pastor joins this process not to provide the proper ending but to encourage people in the telling. Even if the pastor tells the ending to the story that the church has written through the centuries—death, resurrection, and life eternal—mourners must know that they tell and own those endings which are most meaningful to them.

Elements of pastoral care are delivered to the bereaved hospice family in two major ways: through the public ministry of the funeral conducted by the professional minister, and through personal conversations between the pastor or lay caregivers and mourners.

The Funeral

This is the point at which there is an almost inevitable contact between a pastor and a bereaved family. Some of the pastors who were interviewed said that in their experience there is more discussion of funeral plans prior to death in hospice programs than in non-hospice settings. The fact that patients and families are thinking and talking more openly about approaching death enables such discussions.

Sometimes these discussions are initiated by the dying patient, but it is also common for the principal caregiver in the family to bring the subject up. It can be upsetting if the family and the patient are not in agreement on this. Very often in the course of normal hospice care, staff members can support patient or family wishes to talk about funeral plans. Hospice volunteers have frequently gone with patients and families to funeral homes to make the necessary arrangements, even well in advance of the death. Even in situations which do not involve any illness, pre-planning of funerals is becoming increasingly common. Such pre-arrangement by a hospice patient and family does not have to be a morbid occasion. In fact, families often are relieved to have taken care of those details.

One pastor said: "Through hospice care families have become very resource oriented, open to all kinds of resources that will be helpful in their situation. They see very readily that a ritual response to death is a good thing. They recognize, in spite of having lived very close to death for some months, that it is a profound experience, not something to be taken trivially. So they are very appreciative of rituals like the funeral." Interviews seemed to indicate that because of the level of family involvement pastors themselves rarely initiated the pre-arrangement process, unless it was the practice in that particular parish to encourage funeral planning for all its members.

With a few exceptions, it is not unusual for pastors to be asked to conduct funerals for families who have no church affiliation. The experience of a number of hospices is that non-church families tend to ask for a pastor to visit when they begin to plan for a funeral. Some families may merely be superficially satisfying community conventions, but others are acting on their perception that the death of their loved one should be marked with the dignity of a fitting ritual.

Several hospice staffs pointed out that, in their experience, often people who have changed religion or church affiliation revert back to their original church when death approaches. The experience of terminality is so basic that they feel the need to return to a religious context that speaks to them of rootedness. Pastors need to be receptive to such overtures, rather than regarding them cynically or with pious pique.

The funeral offers an opportunity to deal with many needs of the mourners, both in the immediate family and in the larger community. A supportive group is gathered to express the loss which each experiences in his or her own way. Permission is given for people to express their grief in ways that might not be considered appropriate in other settings. The life that has ended is memorialized and recollections are shared. The whole complex of experiences of terminality and death are put in a framework of meaning that comes down across the ages. The funeral communicates that there are ways in which people have found comfort in believing that death is not the end of everything, but that life can begin anew, whether interpreted as life after death for the deceased or life here and tomorrow for the living. The funeral is an integral part of pastoral care to the bereaved, sharing the same objectives as the pastoral conversations with the mourners.[5]

Pastoral Caregiving Conversations

In most instances, the pastor or lay caregiver will have been visiting with the patient and family prior to the death and will continue those visits after the death, to support the family in their mourning. These visits should be (depending, of course, on the wishes of the family) fairly frequent in the early stages of mourning, tapering off over a period of many months.

A sensitive pastor will be aware of the emotionally loaded times of birthdays, anniversaries, and such family-oriented holidays as Thanksgiving, Christmas, and Mother's Day, and make an effort to be in touch with the family at those times. One pastor whose church office has been very inexpensively computerized has put all the significant dates for grieving families of which he is aware into the computer, and gets a weekly print-out of occasions which call for a pastoral response. Even the gathering of the dates from the family in the very early stages of this pastoral care helps to reinforce the remembering process and alerts them to the fact that there will be times when their grieving will take on a special poignancy.

There are occasions when the pastor becomes aware that one particular member of the mourning family has special needs. During her father's illness, Margaret was not able to provide as much help as she would have wished because of her heavy responsibilities as an employed single parent. She felt that she had let her father and mother down. As her pastor ministered to her after her father's death, she was able to verbalize the deep regret she felt. With the pastor and her mother, she came to the insight that her intentions had shown her love for her father, even though circumstances had prevented her active involvement. Later the pastor talked with her about why it had been so difficult for her to resolve the tension between her feeling of failure and her very legitimate responsibilities.

It is not uncommon for other family members to put subtle pressure on a mourner to get over a loss. One pastor talked of a situation in which the adult children had difficulty dealing with their mother's extended grieving. They had all participated in caring for their father before his death. The mother explained, "They all were able to go back to their everyday lives when John died. I don't feel that I had much to go back to. For me life seems empty." The pastoral caregiver's task is not to press the person to conform to expectations, but to respect and support mourning as an individual process.

Most pastors welcome hospice aftercare as a complement to the pastoral care they are giving, acknowledging that family needs are better met through a spectrum of resources. It is in the best interests of parishioners for pastors to collaborate with hospice, just as during the terminal illness, communicating with hospice staff about the ways in which mourning parishioners are dealing with their grief. Such communication is extremely important, also, to prevent people from falling through the cracks, while hospice and the pastor each assume that the other is responding to the needs of the bereaved.

Pastoral Care for the Helpers

One further comment needs to be made before leaving the subject of the bereaved in hospice: Pastors must not be oblivious to the needs of hospice staff, both professional and lay volunteer. A pastor may become acquainted with hospice personnel during the terminal illness of a parishioner, or may have parishioners who are members of a hospice staff. In either instance the pastor should be alert to the mourning of hospice staff members when a patient dies. Because of the number of patients in their caseloads, it is not uncommon for hospice staff to be grieving the loss of three or four patients simultaneously. One must not minimize the attachment that develops very quickly in the deeply sharing and caring relationships of hospice care. These hospice workers need pastoral care as much as bereaved families. The astute pastor will be alert for such needs among hospice workers and provide the same kind of intensive pastoral care to staff as is given to bereaved families.

Summary

The pastoral ministry to bereaved persons, which is as old as the church, is intensified and focused in new ways by the hospice care that has been given to a patient and family during terminal illness. In one sense there is a greater readiness to grieve on the part of parishioners because hospice has schooled them in preparing for death and grief. The pastor must work out a *modus vivendi* for relating to the bereavement aftercare programs of hospice. The pastor must also be alert to the needs of hospice workers whose workloads end up leaving them to grieve for not one, but several hospice patients.

NOTES

1. Glen W. Davidson, ed., *Understanding Mourning* (Minneapolis: Augsburg, 1984), p. 12.

2. Margaretta Bowers et al., *Counseling the Dying* (New York: Aronson, 1981); Richard A. Kalish, *Death, Grief, and Caring Relationships* (Monterey, Calif.: Brooks-Cole, 1981).

3. Ira O. Glick, Robert S. Weiss, and Colin Murray Parkes, *The First Year of Bereavement* (New York: Wiley and Sons, 1974); Davidson, *Understanding Mourning*.

4. Davidson, *Understanding Mourning*, pp. 14-15.

5. Paul E. Irion, *The Funeral and the Mourners* (Nashville: Abingdon Press, 1954, 1979) and *The Funeral: Vestige or Value?* (Nashville: Abingdon Press, 1966; New York: Arno Press, 1976).

CHAPTER 10

HOSPICE AS AN OPPORTUNITY: THE ATTITUDES AND ROLES OF THE PASTOR

Not all hospices are the same. There will be differences in design of the program from community to community, as well as differences in size, budget, and the ways in which they deliver their services. A constant factor in all of the individual varieties, though, is the hospice philosophy, which is codified in the definition provided by the National Hospice Organization. This common feature permits one to generalize with some accuracy about the relationship between hospice and the pastor.

Is hospice an ally, a complement, or a rival? It is probably best to make this judgment first in terms of the hospice concept, and only then in terms of the individual expression of that concept in a particular program. It is historically true that at one time in Western culture the care of the dying was the province of the church. Through the years, the processes of secularization and of the division of labor have widened participation in carrying out many of what were exclusively the church's tasks: law, education, health care, social services—and care of the dying. This, however, does not mean that the church is excluded from any of these functions.

A few pastors interviewed revealed some feelings of competition with hospice, particularly in bereavement aftercare, in spite of the efforts of hospice programs to make clear that they are not trying to become quasi-churches. A secure pastor, one with personal and professional self-knowledge, is open to collaboration with many other helpers in the community. Issues of "turf" are far less important to her or him than the needs of persons.

The attitude of a pastor toward a community agency like hospice will also be influenced by her or his theology of church and ministry. An ecclesiology which defines ministry more closely as activities of the clergy and the church will be less inclined to relate collaboratively with non-ecclesial services. In such a broad view, the church and hospice would run on parallel tracks, only occasionally coming into rivalry.

Most of the pastors contacted viewed hospice as an opportunity for creative ministry by many caregivers, not only the pastor. One pastor said, "Hospice has helped me realize that there are deeply caring people out there; willing to put themselves on the line. This is real Christian charity." Another said, "I see God in the caring of others." The non-defensive stance focuses on the needs of persons and acknowledges that people can use all the help they can get.

The Roles of the Pastor

Because of the clarity of the objectives of hospice care, the role of the pastor in that setting is also clarified. With the exception of the strictly medical treatment of pain and other symptoms, the pastor can be at home in all of hospice's functions. It is highly appropriate for the pastor to be involved in the encouragement of openness in confronting death, in the supportive services to patient and family, in the decision-making processes, and in the bereavement aftercare.

The pastor approaches these functions from the perspective of his or her theological understanding of ministry. But because the hospice mode is inclusive and holistic, each member of the team—professional staff, hospice volunteer, family members, and the pastor—can learn from the others. The single focus of everyone's efforts is to help the patient. The pastor is thoroughly involved in this care, instead of being cordoned off in a sector called "spiritual" or "religious," where he or she is the sole provider of service.

Pastors who were interviewed were asked to characterize their major goal in providing pastoral care in the hospice setting. Some of their responses were "to provide the peace of God and to reduce the fear of the abyss between two lives—now and in the future"; "in word and deed to surround the patient incarnationally with the love of God that can redeem life beyond this suffering"; "to provide dignity to the experience of dying"; "to communicate the 'trustability' of God in a situation of overwhelming change"; "to help families reconnect in a situation where a terrific crisis is tending to disconnect them." It is interesting to note that even with the theological words that some of these statements contain, they describe functions that are appropriate for any person providing hospice care.

A number of pastors described the discomfort they experienced in settings, especially hospitals, where they felt peripheral to the structure and were unclear of what was expected from them. These same pastors said that hospice, rather than making them feel alien, drew them into the caregiving in ways that made their functions clearer. A number of roles are open to the pastor in this setting: companion, spiritual caregiver, theologian-in-residence, pastoral counselor, priest.

1. The Role of Companion

Some of the literature growing out of the revived interest in spiritual direction makes considerable use of the concept of "companioning." A similar note is present in the common theme of being a "presence" to someone. The thought of a pastor standing with a parishioner is nothing new.

One pastor put it thus: "It is easy to make contact with their loneliness. Their hunger for meaning comes out into the open if they are given a chance to talk." The experience of dying, as has been pointed out, is isolating, because the dying person is approaching the imminent ending of life, while all those near to him or her go on living. No amount of intimacy in relationship can change this fact. But having caring persons who are close can mitigate the loneliness.

Some clergy will find encouragement in the words of John Hinton:

> The priest has a more traditional and, for some people, an essential part to play in preparing a person for death. As minister . . . he can give great comfort to the dying patient. . . . He can speak with greater authority to the dying and assure him that whatever happens after this life ends, God will be there to receive him, perhaps asserting that the Lord is forgiving.[1]

Another approach was described by one of the pastors interviewed. He said, "Knowing that they are talking with a minister makes the conversation implicitly religious. They bring God in, I don't. God is 'found' in relationships."

These two approaches suggest that the model of companioning has three elements: being present to the person, listening, and speaking. It might be proposed that this order is normative, that speaking should come only after presence is established and one has heard carefully what the dying person is saying. The quality of relationship is of utmost importance. Here hospice involvement is a benefit because of its focus on relating as essential in dealing with death.

Unless there is a history of a disastrous experience with the clergy, many people are open to a pastoral relationship. They believe that the pastor is concerned about their well-being and wants to do everything he or she can to offer comfort and strength to the dying person. The pastor is not only a person, but also a representative of the church, of which the patient may be a committed member or which may be one of the links to a stability remembered from the past. The interest and concern of the pastor and the loneliness of the patient are usually enough to open doors, permitting the relationship to move readily to some depth.

From the interviews with pastors a number of ways to establish a relationship with the dying patient were cited. One pastor said, "I begin talking about the concerns of the patient for his or her family rather than for self when starting the relationship with the patient. Then, later, we move to talking about the patient and his or her needs." This pastor found such an approach developed openness more readily, because the person felt more comfortable talking about others' needs before discussing his or her own.

Another pastor wrote of a series of questions that he explores in visits with the hospice patient. These are not ticked off in questionnaire fashion but provide the structure for a whole series of pastoral conversations. Whether or not the questions originated with him, they are an extremely valuable resource for establishing a relationship with the hospice patient. Of course, these questions would be approached in a slightly different way with a parishioner whom one knew very well, but they generally would pertain to any pastoral relationship.

The questions include "How long have you been ill?" "How ill are you?" "How were you told what you have?" "How did you feel about the way in which you were told?" "What does this illness mean to you?" "How has the illness changed you?" "How has the illness changed those around you?" "Who has been most helpful to you?" "Do you have fears?" "What are you putting into this experience?" Again, it must be emphasized that such questions are not asked as if the pastor were making a survey. Rather, they suggest directions conversations can take over the course of a number of visits. There is no magic in their wording, but note how they penetrate to the deeper levels of the person's experience.

The important elements in establishing the relationship are to indicate concern, to communicate that the patient retains a large measure of control over the relationship, and to demonstrate that the pastor is willing to go to any depth the patient wishes. One needs to recall that hospice care is given in unhurried fashion, conveying a willingness to take all the time the patient wishes for relating. Of course, quantity is not a substitute for quality, but anything that resembles the perfunctory obviously will be out of focus with the complete picture of hospice care.

2. The Role of Spiritual Caregiver

While this is not the responsibility solely of the pastor, it is a function for which the pastor is accountable. However, it can be understood in a variety of ways, ranging from closely defined to broadly understood.

Close definition of spiritual caregiving includes specifically priestly acts, administration of sacraments, prayers, Scripture reading, and talking about explicitly religious or theological concerns: theodicy, sin, forgiveness, salvation, and eternal life. These are all perfectly valid elements of spiritual caregiving.

Broader definitions would include probing for the meaning of the mysterious processes of living and dying, and would recognize that not everyone will approach that quest through traditional religious beliefs, concepts, or language. One pastor was talking about this kind of spiritual caregiving when she said, "The work of the pastor flows into more of the patient's life than just 'God-talk' and 'churchiness.'" Nor is this simply a one-way street, for the pastor can also learn from participating in the patient's struggle for meaning.

Every pastor develops his or her own style of spiritual caregiving based on how he or she defines it. Working within a hospice program certainly does tend to support the broader definition, that is, not limiting one's service to traditional religious concepts. The needs of the patient and family are instead foremost in determining the care that is given. The pastor who is comfortable working in terms of the broader definition will more adequately represent the breadth of the hospice approach in responding to the spectrum of needs of particular patients.

Hospice supports patients in determining their own agendas for dealing with death. This extends to spiritual caregiving. The pastor is not expected to come up with answers for questions that are not being asked, nor to press the patient toward a particular point of view. If one is truly "with" a patient, empathically as well as spatially, the person's belief system, however conventional or unconventional, begins to emerge. The effective spiritual caregiver will not immediately press that system into a normative form but will draw the person out to say just what these personal truths and values mean in the present situation.

Margarett Schlientz suggests that there are a number of issues that emerge in spiritual care. These include attitudes toward life, the meaning of suffering, and assessment of relationships which provide strength, religious beliefs, and experiences of forgiveness.[2] According to the way people handle these issues and proceeding from their own experience, they draw a line beyond which the quality of life is no longer acceptable. This delineation makes a statement about the life of this person, which involves his or her sense of self-worth, of strength, of accomplishment.

Where this line is drawn is to some extent dependent upon the quality of the patient's relationships with others. One gets a sense of whether the patient feels strength flowing from other persons into his or her life, or feels strength being drained away by others. The patient will also reflect on the care being given and received. Many patients speak of being overwhelmed by the gracious care, the love beyond measure they are receiving. Other persons will reflect on relationships that have been disappointing and look for reconciliation as a way of bringing quality to life.

The situation of approaching death usually causes the patient's understanding of the meaning of suffering to be included in her or his picture of life. The source of suffering may be explored as well as the means by which one copes with suffering. Many patients do not feel that they are coping as well as they might in this situation. Their sense of failure supports a negative self-image; they chide themselves for not emerging triumphantly from their suffering. The sensitive spiritual caregiver will provide support for what they are able to do.

Patients may also want to discuss specific religious beliefs, such as, the efficacy of prayer, the place of faith in dealing with crisis, the meaning of hope for new life. At times the patient's questions are requests for clarification or explanation; at other times they are the probings of doubt. The spiritual caregiver has to guard against prematurely closing discussion of such issues by providing ready-made answers or by being critical of questioning and doubt. One has to put aside older, mechanistic understandings of the need for dying persons to achieve the right beliefs or to profess some particular faith statement. Such understandings have often been warrants for forcing a person toward resolution of a faith issue, under the urgency of approaching death. A more sensitive pastoral response is to see value in the questing person, not only in the person with ready answers.

The very helpful article by Beresford sums it up:

> Simply, hospice spiritual care is "being" with the patient and family, not necessarily "doing" any specific tasks other than compassionate, active listening. . . .
> Ideally, the caregiver comes without an agenda or a specific spiritual message or answer and on the patient's terms, whatever the patient's wishes, beliefs or questions—if any.[3]

The traditional role of the pastor in relating to the dying person is preparing the patient to die. The assumption was that there were certain words or acts that had to be said or done by the patient before he or she could die in a state of grace. In this model, the pastoral caregiver felt a sense of urgency about "saving" the patient.

The more dynamic understandings of faith and grace in contemporary theology put more attention on the process of relationship than on the mechanical performance of a particular act. The goal of the pastoral caregiver is to help the person to an experience of acceptance, in any or all dimensions, from acceptance by a caring person to acceptance by the transcendent. Mills writes:

> They [clergy] feel obliged to be available, to offer
> relationship and sustenance [to the dying]. They hope
> that persons will avail themselves of the offer and
> come to terms with their life and death. Deep down
> they may wish that persons die believing. But the
> belief they covet for the dying person is not so much in
> this or that creed or confession as it is in the triumph of
> love and hope and meaning over death.[4]

This dynamic, general understanding of preparing
persons to die fits well into the holistic hospice
approach. All of the efforts of hospice are focused on
preparing a person to die. The pastoral caregiver is
one of the operative elements in that function, but
certainly not the only one. Again, the breadth of
understanding of the hospice approach helps in
clarifying the pastoral task.

Most pastors accept the responsibility to comfort the
dying. We need to be reminded of the root of that
word. "Comfort" meant originally "to make strong."
It is not soothing or sedating by ignoring death and
jumping ahead to the hope of heaven. Pastoral care
operates where people are, in the midst of the
experience of dying and separating. It empathizes
with the pain and anguish, the guilt and anxiety, that
may be experienced by the patient and family. It
encourages people to talk about these experiences
openly and to move beyond them to a measure of
acceptance—to envision death, one way or another, as
more than waste or obliteration. The pastoral caregiver is a companion and guide in this struggle,
knowing that he or she is caught up in the same
mortality.

Sometimes, in preparing to die, people have an
agenda of unfinished business that they would like to
resolve. They are aware of disruptions in relationships, of failures to maintain earlier commitments, of
estrangement from earlier values or faith. They want

to express their regret and to seek some kind of restoration, if possible. The pastor does not have an obligation to induce such an agenda, but when it is apparent that the person wants to talk about an unresolved issue in personal or religious life, the pastor is open to respond. Sometimes direct restoration of relationships is possible. In other instances the passage of years has brought such changes that only a symbolic restoration can be made. Either way, the person can experience some resolution and feel a new readiness to face approaching death.

Rudolf Otto conceptualized the experience of the holy in two ways, the *Mysterium Tremendum* and *Mysterium Fascinans*, the mixture of awe and fascination.[5] Even very traditional theological formulations that describe the love and the justice of God mirror this ambiguity. Psychological and sociological studies described by Feifel, of the correlation between religious faith and attitudes toward dying, show a similar ambiguity.[6] While one might expect strong religious faith to remove all fear of dying, such faith, particularly when it emphasizes the judgment of God, can also produce significant anxiety.

The pastoral caregiver has to be aware of the possible existence of this ambiguity in the feeling and thinking of the patient. Only if the patient is free to talk about his or her vision of the transcendent is there the possibility of exploration of both sides of the paradox. Again, providing an opportunity for the patient rather than the pastor to do the talking is clearly valuable.

The point at which this becomes real to the patient is in relating. Abstract discussions of the nature of God are far less helpful than exploration of the subjective dimensions of relating to the transcendent. What is the person feeling: awe, mystery, silence, unconditional acceptance, conditional love, fear, anger, belongingness, isolation, peace, guilt? How does the person picture the relationship: adversarial, parental, rescuing, supporting? What response is the person making in the relationship: commitment, passive dependency, acquiescence, defiance? It is obvious that the person has to take the lead in such discussion, with the pastor functioning as an enabler, a catalyst. Such a model of pastoral caregiving is supported by the hospice philosophy of giving people the right to die in their own way, rather than forcing them to conform to a pattern set by an outside authority.

One pastor said, "I try to help people see God coming to us, rather than pursuing God." This is a way of obviating any patient compulsions to develop a certain kind of relationship with the transcendent. It tries to free people from the driving need to achieve a certain state. It helps patients see God as present in the affairs of living and dying, and sharpens their perceptions of belongingness.

The radical termination of life as we know it is difficult, if not impossible, to accept fully. So it is very common to think in terms of some ongoing existence after death. Such concepts of the afterlife cannot be empirically based but are articles of personal faith. Some will use the words and symbols of Scripture and speak in terms of personal survival in heaven or eternity; others will think in terms of individual cessation but social or biological immortality. Because the life-death continuum is not directly known but is a mystery, it is only natural that people have many questions about life after death.

These questions take two general forms: What is the nature of life after death? and, Will I live after death? The nature of life after death has to be described metaphorically. Some of the metaphors are used to describe hoped-for continuity with present life.

Personal identity and relationships continue on, described in terms of recognition and reunion. Metaphors of completion and fulfillment describe ways in which life after death continues this life in a perfected state: life with God, relief from pain, peace, purification, reward, release, rest. Still other metaphors describe discontinuity with present life. The life after death is characterized by freedom from finite limitation, by being no longer subject to time and space, by entering a new realm of existence, by being accepted into the whole.

The other question—Will I live after death—depends on how judgment figures in the picture. For those who think in Platonic terms, immortality of the soul is a standard human endowment. But those who think of life after death as a gift from God, as in the Christian concept of resurrection, believe that it may or may not be given. The thought of judgment impinges here and a person may wonder, Will I be found worthy? Christian thought has traditionally divided between those who propose a universalism in which everyone is given new life by the love of God, and those who hold to a process of election by which new life is given only to some.

Patients and family members will be in one of two modes as they talk about life after death. In the affirming mode, they have either accepted the teaching of others or have worked out their own responses to their questions about this mystery, so they are able to state their belief affirmatively. Those in the questioning mode probe what life after death might mean for them. They may find that earlier conceptualizations are no longer satisfying. They struggle to state their hope in new ways.

In either mode the pastoral caregiver supports whatever affirmations individuals can make. The concern is not so much for people to have a "correct" understanding but that they have an understanding that satisfies their personal quest. If we *knew* the truth, it would be different. Pastors need to acknowledge with intellectual humility that we deal here with a mystery. Pastoral honesty and integrity requires that one respond to questions with "I can't know absolutely, but this is what I believe . . ." or "I have found it helpful to think about it this way . . ." or "Through the centuries the church has taught and believed that . . ." But even more important is to ask the person what he or she thinks or believes.

A second crucial step is to help the patient or family member reflect on what that particular understanding does for her or him. This is not done in an effort to discount or devalue a particular interpretation, but to help the person understand why that interpretation is helpful in dealing with the situation of terminality.

If the pastoral caregiver can accept the hospice's commitment to allow people to die in their own way, in the way most satisfying to them, then it should also be possible to let people work through to their own interpretations of death and its aftermath and find a belief, an understanding, that most deeply satisfies their own needs for meaning. This may represent for some a sizable deviation from their regular pattern of trying to get assent for "correct" doctrine, but it is a direct outgrowth of the dedication of hospice to allowing people to die their own deaths.

3. The Role of Theologian-in-Residence

Not only is the pastor a supportive caregiver, she or he is also a theologian-in-residence in the hospice situation. These two functions are closely related. Not only is the pastoral caregiver theologically motivated, the pastor is also skilled in reflecting theologically on life situations. This is a service to both the hospice patient and family and to the church.

Employing the theme of Seward Hiltner's time-

honored book, *Preface to Pastoral Theology*, the pastor
not only applies theological teachings to life situations
but also uses life situations as the basis for theologizing.[7] More than one pastor interviewed affirmed that
experience with hospice patients and families had put
them more in touch with their own theologies. The
questions people ask, the resources upon which they
draw for help, the ways in which they discover
meaning in living and dying, constitute powerful data
for theologizing.

In discussions with pastors about their theological
reflection on the situations of hospice patients, a
recurring theme was incarnation. They told of ways
patients had talked with them about their sense that
God was with them in their dying: in the loving care
they were receiving, in the supportive relationships
which sustained them, in their hope. The sense of
"Emmanuel" provided a context of belonging that
relieved the painful sense of isolation their illness had
brought. Immanence took on a new meaning.
Theology itself was taken from the realm of the
abstract and put into the context of real living and
dying.

Another unavoidable theological issue in the situation of terminality involves the meaning of the
statement, "It is God's will." Any pastor is familiar with
the tension of ideas that arises as soon as one takes the
theological proposition that God is omnipotent and
relates it to a particular human situation, particularly to
a tragic one. If God has willed this illness, is it
punishment, is it testing? How can a good, loving God
cause such suffering? As Beresford points out,

> Often the patient asks "why me?" "why now?" or
> "what happens when I die?" The spiritual caregiver
> basically answers "I don't know," acknowledging that
> these are indeed good, hard questions and encourag-
> ing the patient to make his or her own spiritual
> explorations.[8]

The ability to take such an approach depends on how one defines being a theologian. If it is defined as having the answers, which are in turn transmitted to another person, then such an open-ended conversation would seem like failure. On the other hand, if being a theologian is focused more on a process of questing with others than on having prefabricated answers, the approach described by Beresford enables people to seek their own answers. Like any good teacher, the pastor guides the process by sharpening questions, exploring implications, and explaining the answers others have found in the past. But the patient retains the responsibility to find those answers that are most personally meaningful. Such an approach is strongly supported by the hospice philosophy, which frees a person from an authority structure that does not permit the freedom to work out one's own pattern of dying.

Similarly, just as hospice personnel are not invulnerable to their own mortality, to loss and grief, the theologian-in-residence is not invulnerable to doubts and frustration about not having answers come easily. Hospice staff members have to have support systems to help them cope with their vulnerabilities—pastors do too. They can learn that they do not have to have all the answers, that it is understandable that their faith weakens and wavers when stressed by tragedy. Hospice workers find that they can serve patients and families better, more empathically, if they are willing to admit these vulnerabilities and to cope with them. Pastors who honestly face their own doubts and questions, their own "theological feelings," can understand better the struggles of patients for faith. They are more likely to join patients in their quests for theological meaning than to provide answers, to argue with patient's views, or to reject people with whom they do not agree.

Meaning, theological or otherwise, is not only achieved through cognition—knowing ideas or facts. It is also rooted in a perception of one's place in the order of things. Meaning is found in relational knowledge—knowing as I am known. Life has meaning when we have a sense of personal worth because we know that we belong—to one who loves us, to a family, to a church, to the universe, to God. The theologian-in-residence functions as much in relatedness as in the area of intellectual cognition.

4. The Role of Pastoral Counselor

It is clear that we are not describing a list of functions of the spiritual caregiver in hospice as much as a series of perspectives for understanding what the giver of pastoral care is and does. The task is rather constant: to help people die with grace, to help people mourn with grace. This task can be approached with equal helpfulness from a number of perspectives, each appropriate to the self-understanding of the caregiver or to the way needs are perceived in the situation. The pastoral counseling approach suggests that the pastor will spend considerable time with the patient or family member, working through a specific problem or issue.

If one assumes the role of pastoral counselor, a primary task is reality testing. Effective counseling proceeds on the basis of clarifying the reality in which the patient lives. If reality is badly skewed, it is difficult for the person or the counselor to work toward development of coping mechanisms.

Reality testing is especially active in the hospice setting; this is another instance in which being related to hospice care facilitates the pastor's caregiving. The reality is that the patient is in all probability dying. (One always has to recognize, though, that there is the rare exception of the hospice patient who does not die when expected.) This reality has substantial objective support in the diagnosis and prognosis reached through the physician's observations and testing or surgical exploration. In time the declining condition of the patient may become apparent even to the non-medical observer. A consensus develops that the patient is dying. This is explained to the patient and family, but, as has been pointed out earlier, acceptance of that reality is usually ambivalent—and not without reason on their part, however slim. Hospice acknowledges and respects the psychological defenses of those who are most closely involved, even though it does not concur with them. Hospice staff members, without attacking anyone's defenses, proceed to act on the basis of their perception of the reality of the situation for "99.44 percent" of the patients. Hospice simply serves the patient as one who is dying.

Pastoral counseling operates in a similar mode. It certainly must begin with the reality perceived by the patient. It neither ignores nor argues with that perception; the counselor continues to function, with equal legitimacy, on the basis of her or his own perception of reality. This is done empathically, without condescension.

Death, like life, is mysterious, inscrutable, and, as such, is fearsome. The unknown is understandably frightening. This is seen in the difficulty humans have in dealing with approaching death. Some denial or resistance is very common, because death creates some fear, no matter how natural it is.

Several of the pastors interviewed had seen people whose wish for pastoral care seemed motivated by fear. "Many patients I have seen, especially those without much church connection, are motivated by fear. They want to cover their options. It is the old foxhole religion. I know one instance where remission occurred and the family dropped away from the church."

Other instances show people, even though they may originally be motivated by fear, finding new levels of commitment in crisis situations. As Gordon Allport points out in his concept of "functional autonomy," motives can change in time and what was once caused by relatively inferior motivation can in a new situation be produced by more helpful motives.[9] For example, the student who gets good grades simply to please parents may gradually come to do good work out of intellectual curiosity and the love of learning.

John Hinton writes that dying persons with a strong religious faith, or those patients without any significant religious faith, had less anxiety than those with a limited faith commitment which found little expression in their lives.[10] The lack of integrity of such a position apparently increases the anxiety of the dying person. Some of this is due to the fact that the faith commitment is so superficial that it is an insufficient resource for coping with crisis. Or the fear may be produced by the expectation of judgment for one's insincerity.

The pastoral counselor in the hospice setting will be alert for expressions of anxiety or fear in patients and family members. They will be encouraged to express these feelings in a context of understanding and acceptance. The pastor, functioning as counselor, will have an ally in the hospice staff, who all have been giving the same encouragement too. One pastor said: "I have found hospice patients more articulate in expressing their feelings. The hospice staff has helped them to 'name the demons.' Patients tend to talk more about what they are going through. This gives the pastor more freedom; someone has broken the ground, and people let their feelings surface."

The natural tendency in conversation is to minimize such negative emotions as fear, to divert to more pleasant thoughts and feelings. This does little to enable release from fear. The goal of pastoral counseling for the hospice patient is not to remove all fear. That is highly unlikely to happen. The goal is to keep fear within manageable limits by making it as specific as possible, which will suggest ways of coping with the fear. For instance, fear of isolation and loneliness can be dealt with by providing a good deal of support; fear of suffering can be met by pain control. Other fears, such as the fear of meaninglessness, or of the ending of consciousness, or of separation from loved ones after death, are more pervasive. Simply countering these with a theological statement or with the telling of the biblical story is the effort of an observer to solve the problem. Actually, any relief from these deep fears has to come from an affirming process within the patient himself or herself. The person needs the help of a sensitive counselor in exploring deep inner resources of faith. Anything less than such a process is a superficial treatment for a profound problem.

The traditional linking of mortality and sin in Judeo-Christian theology has deeply influenced Western thought, even below the levels of consciousness. Even without making a straight line, cause-and-effect connection between sin and death, the summative nature of the experience of dying causes a review of life that is bound to contain elements of regret for neglected opportunities, for alienations, for actions which run contrary to one's values.

One spiritual caregiver told of working with a patient who had great difficulty confronting the fact that she was dying until she confided that she was still dealing with a great deal of guilt over an abortion she had had twenty years before. Until she had some way of dealing with that guilt, she could not let loose of life.

Because life's relationships are rarely totally positive, disruptions and estrangements occur, leaving a residue of pain and unresolved feelings. It is not uncommon for dying patients to deal with their regret or guilt over such alienation by trying to find some way to make things right. Sometimes they look for actual, practical measures that they can take to right a wrong. In other instances, they work for an improvement of attitudes leading to reconciliation.

Several pastors interviewed spoke of this situation, described by one of their number: "I see people in obvious tension—hoping for death, feeling guilty because of that hope." This feeling has different points of origin for different people. Some feel they are "playing God" by willing life to end; some feel they are failing to affirm the value of living; some feel they are violating the social value of "not giving up"; some feel that their families will think they are being deliberately abandoned. Any of these interpretations of the wish to die can cause a person to experience guilt.

Even though we have become accustomed to differentiating guilt feelings from real guilt, there needs to be recognition that from a phenomenological point of view all guilt is real to the person experiencing it. To say, "You don't have to feel guilty about that," may offer very little comfort. It is far more effective to help the person explore why he or she feels the guilt. Sometimes this will lead to the person recognizing that he or she is taking on guilt for something for which he or she is not responsible. At other times the person will be able to describe real personal accountability, to desire to correct what can be corrected, and to seek forgiveness for what cannot be undone.

It is not the responsibility of the pastoral counselor in the hospice setting to induce such expression of guilt. The pressure to stimulate deathbed confessions fortunately passed with the emergence of more dynamic theological understandings of the human situation. The notion of having to die with a clean slate expired with the mechanistic understandings of sin and forgiveness held by past generations: that one must take the specific steps of feeling convicted and of repenting of a particular misdeed before one could be assured of forgiveness. Human motivations are so complex that any such models quickly fall victim to oversimplification. It is far more effective to begin where the person is and to respond to evident needs and wishes.

Certainly terminal illness has all the ingredients for being regarded as a crisis. David Switzer points to several indicators that a crisis is present: The problem is of fairly recent origin; the situation of the person is deteriorating; the person no longer feels capable of coping.[11] He also reminds us that crisis lies in the person, not in the situation; two persons may respond very differently to the same problem. One may be able to confront and deal with it; the other may feel totally powerless to do anything. Only the latter person is in crisis.

Pastors ministering in a hospice situation need to assess whether or not a crisis exists for the patient or family members. If so, crisis counseling is an appropriate mode for spiritual caregiving, helping them to explore their situation, the resources for dealing with it, and to take some action to cope and to get past the feeling of being powerless and ineffectual.

Walter Johnson speaks of "blossoming in times of crisis" and is quoted by Beresford:

> Some of the signs of this blossoming may include an expanded range of emotional expression; a deeper sense of bondedness with self, others and with the world; an expanded sense of meaning; and expanded coping power; a feeling of being in command of the situation despite the disease; a wider range of choices; a growing capacity for love; a sense of humor and an apparent sense of inner calm.[12]

Although one needs to take care not to overly romanticize this notion, Pollyanna fashion, it does point to the way in which people can work through what has become for them the crisis of approaching death and loss. One pastor described his approach as helping people to ask, "What can give me strength to get through this crisis? How did I get through crisis in the past?"

Hospice care and the philosophy which guides it fit very well the pattern of crisis counseling. The openness and honesty encouraged by hospice help people to define and understand their situations and the threats they contain. Hospice rests heavily on supportive relationships and provides a panoply of resources to help people cope with their needs. It encourages active involvement in dealing with the problem rather than passive hand-wringing. It continues to support as people master new attitudes and behaviors that enable them to feel some control over their situation.

One pastor said, "Through hospice I have learned to understand the dynamics of families in crisis. Not only have I become more knowledgeable, but I have more sensitive awareness of the intricacies of family relationships and the feelings they generate. I have to minister to each individual and to all of them collectively as well." So pastoral care in a hospice situation can easily develop into a form of family counseling.

5. The Role of Priest

The priestly functions of the pastoral caregiver are also very much involved in hospice care. The administration of sacraments and conducting other rituals appropriate for the care of the dying and the grieving are a part of pastoral responsibility. These priestly acts are highly effective in providing meaning and in conveying a sense of vital belongingness. The gathering of a family for receiving the eucharist together with the dying patient, the funeral which marks the ending of a life and the ongoingness of new life, the prayers of the community of faith, can all be powerful experiences of solidarity and caring and support.

Other priestly acts are less familiar in some churches. There is growing use of brief services for the commendation of the dying, which were formerly found mainly in high liturgical tradition. One pastor described his experience: "I have been criticized by some parishioners for offering commendation of the dying when a person was very near death. They interpreted it as pushing the person to die, sort of hastening her death. But the family was overjoyed to have the service. It was a way for them to give permission for the patient to let go, a very satisfying closure." Even the Roman Catholic church has moved away from the idea of "last rites," which had become a kind of negative signal that the end was near. Commendation of the dying, whether it follows a formal pattern or simply takes the form of extempore prayer, is a ritual that marks the dignified conclusion of a life and the beginning of the separation of bereavement.

Another priestly act which can be a meaningful part of the care of hospice patients and their families is confession. Although most churches in the Protestant tradition do not have rituals beyond prayers of general confession, the theological differences in Christendom have not involved confession per se, but absolution and penance. When the parishioner wishes to talk confessionally, the pastor will be open to that conversation. It is not something to which the person should be compelled; it is most effective when voluntary.

There always has to be a careful distinction made

between efficacious rituals and magic. One of the best ways of describing this difference is to see effective ritual as strengthening a person to encounter and transcend a great difficulty, while magic is understood as a way of escaping from the dire straits of crisis. There are times when people, without really understanding what they are asking, want the pastor to be a magician. The pastor's function then becomes not to scold or reject them but to help them explore their expectation and the feelings of desperation and anxiety that stir it.

Many rituals, such as eucharist, anointing and prayers, are seen by some patients and families as potentially healing. The pastor sometimes questions if such rites are requested as part of a pattern of denial of the reality of approaching death. In fact, they have a built-in ambiguity which enables them to be understood either as pathways to healing or preparation for dying. These can both be valid expectations, as long as the ambiguity is not resolved. One Roman Catholic hospice patient and his priest prayed often that a healing miracle would occur. As the patient's condition deteriorated drastically, the priest began to pray for the "miracle beyond death," picking up the tension of the ambiguity.

Summary

The role that the pastoral caregiver takes has two points of origin, the pastor's own self-understanding and the perceived needs of the patient and family. The roles which have been described here are not mutually exclusive. They suggest, rather, a number of ways to be effective in responding to the needs of the dying and the grieving.

There is a timeworn sermon illustration that tells of an old church which had carved in the stone on the inside of the pulpit the words, "Preach as a dying man to dying men." In spite of the archaic, non-inclusive language, these words set the theme for spiritual caregiving in the hospice setting. Any role, any pastoral or priestly function, any caring response to a need, is founded on common human mortality, enabling the ultimate empathy.

NOTES

1. John Hinton, *Dying* (Baltimore: Penguin Books, 1967), p. 124.
2. Larry Beresford, "Spiritual Care in Hospice," *California Hospice Report* 2, no. 7 (Dec. 1984): 12.
3. Ibid., p. 4.
4. Liston O. Mills, "Issues for the Clergy in the Care of the Dying and Bereaved," in *Dying and Death*, ed. David Barton (Baltimore: Williams & Wilkins, 1977), p. 205.
5. Rudolf Otto, *The Idea of the Holy*, trans. J. W. Harvey (London: Oxford University Press, 1928).
6. Herman Feifel, "Religious Conviction and Fear of Death among the Healthy and the Terminally Ill," in *Death and Identity*, rev. ed., ed. Robert Fulton (Bowie, Md.: Charles Press Publishers, 1976), pp. 120-30.
7. Seward Hiltner, *Preface to Pastoral Theology* (Nashville: Abingdon Press, 1958), pp. 20ff.
8. Beresford, "Spiritual Care," p. 4.
9. Gordon W. Allport, *Pattern and Growth in Personality* (New York: Holt, Rinehart, and Winston, 1961), pp. 219ff.
10. Hinton, *Dying*, p. 83.
11. David Switzer, *The Minister as Crisis Counselor*, rev. ed. (Nashville: Abingdon Press, 1986), chapter 2. See also Howard Stone, *Crisis Counseling* (Philadelphia: Fortress Press, 1976).
12. Beresford, "Spiritual Care," pp. 12-13.

BIBLIOGRAPHY

BOOKS

Ainsworth-Smith, Ian, and Speck, Peter. *Letting Go*. London: SPCK, 1983.

Barton, David, ed. *Dying and Death*. Baltimore: Williams & Wilkins, 1977.

Bowers, Margaretta et al. *Counseling the Dying*. New York: Aronson, 1981.

Brim, Orville G. et al. *The Dying Patient*. New York: Russell Sage Foundation Books, 1970.

Caughill, Rita E. *The Dying Patient: A Supportive Approach*. New York: Little, Brown, 1976.

Chirhan, John T., ed. *Coping with Death and Dying: An Interdisciplinary Approach*. Lanham, Md.: University Press of America, 1985.

Corr, Charles A., and Corr, Donna M. *Hospice Care*. New York: Springer, 1983.

Cousins, Norman. *The Anatomy of an Illness as Perceived by the Patient: Reflections on Healing and Regeneration*. New York: W. W. Norton, 1979.

Davidson, Glen W., ed. *The Hospice: Development and Administration*. 2nd ed. Washington: Hemisphere Publishing Corp., 1985.

_____. *Living with Dying*. Minneapolis: Augsburg, 1975.

_____. *Understanding Mourning*. Minneapolis: Augsburg, 1984.

Dobihal, Edward F., Jr., and Stewart, Charles William. *When a Friend Is Dying*. Nashville: Abingdon Press, 1984.

Dubois, Paul M. *The Hospice Way of Death*. New York: Human Sciences Press, 1979.

Bibliography

Dulany, Joseph P. *We Can Minister with the Dying.* Nashville: Discipleship Resources, 1987.

Fulton, Robert. *Death and Identity.* Bowie, Md.: Charles Press, 1976.

Glick, Ira O.; Weiss, Robert S.; and Parkes, Colin Murray. *The First Year of Bereavement.* New York: John Wiley and Sons, 1974. Bowie, Md.: Charles Press, 1976.

Hamilton, Michael P., and Reid, Helen, eds. *A Hospice Handbook.* Grand Rapids: Eerdmans, 1980.

Hinton, John. *Dying.* Baltimore: Penguin Books, 1967.

Irion, Paul E. *The Funeral and the Mourners.* Nashville: Abingdon Press, 1966.

————. *The Funeral: Vestige or Value?* Nashville: Abingdon Press, 1966. New York: Arno Press, 1976.

Kalish, Richard A. *Death, Grief, and Caring Relationships.* Monterey, Calif.: Brooks-Cole, 1981.

————, ed. *Caring Relationships: The Dying and the Bereaved.* Perspectives on Death and Dying Series. Farmingdale, N.Y.: Baywood, 1980.

Kübler-Ross, Elisabeth. *On Death and Dying.* New York: Macmillan, 1969.

Kutscher, Austin et al., eds. *Hospice U.S.A.* Foundation of Thanatology Series. New York: Columbia University Press, 1983.

Lamerton, Richard. *Care of the Dying.* Westport: Technomic Publishing Company, 1976.

Munley, Anne. *The Hospice Alternative.* New York: Basic Books, 1983.

National Hospice Organization. *Standards of a Hospice Program of Care.* Arlington, Va.: National Hospice Organization, 1979, 1982.

Oates, Wayne E., and Oates, Charles E. *People in Pain: Guidelines for Pastoral Care.* Philadelphia: Westminster Press, 1985.

Pacholski, R. A., and Corr, C. A., eds. *New Directions in Death Education and Counseling.* Arlington, Va.: Forum for Death Education and Counseling, 1981.

Parkes, Colin Murray. *Bereavement: Studies of Grief in Adult Life.* New York: International Universities Press, 1972.

Pattison, E. Mansell. *The Experience of Dying.* Englewood Cliffs, N.J.: Prentice-Hall, 1977.

Platt, Nancy. *Pastoral Care to the Cancer Patient.* Springfield, Ill.: Thomas, 1980.

Raven, Ronald W., ed. *The Dying Patient.* Tunbridge Wells, England: Pitman Medical, 1975.

Richards, Larry, and Johnson, Paul. *Death and the Caring Community.* Portland: Multnomah Press, 1980.

Simonton, Carl. *Getting Well Again: A Step-by-Step Self-Help Guide to Overcoming Cancer for Patients and Their Families.* Los Angeles: Jeremy P. Tarcher, 1978.

Society for the Right to Die. *The Physician and the Hopelessly Ill Patient.* New York: Society for the Right to Die, 1985.

Stone, Howard. *Crisis Counseling.* Philadelphia: Fortress Press, 1976.

Switzer, David. *The Minister as Crisis Counselor.* Rev. ed. Nashville: Abingdon Press, 1986.

Wentzel, Kenneth B. *To Those Who Need It Most, Hospice Means Hope.* Boston: Charles River Books, 1981.

ARTICLES

Beresford, Larry. "Spiritual Care in Hospice." *California Hospice Report* 2, no. 7. (Dec. 1984): 1-16.

Berman, Alan L. "Belief in Afterlife, Religion, Religiosity, and Life-Threatening Experience." *Omega* 5, no. 2 (1974): 127-35.

Cairns, Alexander B., and Hunter, James S. "Similarities and Differences of Care in a Medical Center." *The Journal of Pastoral Care* 40, no. 1 (Mar. 1986): 68-75.

Herman Feifel. "Religious Conviction and Fear of Death among the Healthy and the Terminally Ill." *Journal for the Scientific Study of Religion* 13, no. 3 (Sept. 1974): 353-60.

Gates, George N. "Where Is the Pastoral Counselor in the Hospice Movement?" *The Journal of Pastoral Care* 61, no. 1 (Mar. 1987): 32-39.

Greer, David S., and Mor, Vincent. "How Medicare Is Altering the Hospice Movement." *Hastings Center Report* 15, no. 5 (Oct. 1985): 5-9.

Edward J. Holland, "The Art of Hospice Spiritual Care." Unpublished essay.

Lester, David. "Religious Behavior and Fear of Death." *Omega* 2 (1970): 181-88.

Lifton, Robert Jay. "The Politics of Immortality." *Psychology Today* (Nov. 1970): 70-73, 108-10.

Longsworth, William M. "At the Edge of Death: A Pastor's Role in Decisions about Withholding and Withdrawing Treatment." *Perkins Journal* 39 (Jan. 1986): 44-50.

Reeves, Robert B., Jr. "Professionalism and Compassion in the Care of the Dying." *Pastoral Psychology* 22 (1971): 7-14.

Saunders, Cicely. "Telling Patients." *District Nursing* (Sept. 1965): 145-54.

Tehan, Claire. "Has Success Spoiled Hospice?" *Hastings Center Report* 15, no. 5 (Oct. 1985): 10-13.

INDEX

Index